Ageless Beauty the Natural Way

Anita Guyton

Thorsons
An Imprint of HarperCollins*Publishers*

D0170365

Thorsons
An Imprint of HarperCollins*Publishers*
77–85 Fulham Palace Road,
Hammersmith, London W6 8JB

Published by Thorsons 1993
10 9 8 7 6 5 4 3 2 1

Anita Guyton assets the moral right to
be identified as the author of this work

A catalogue record for this book
is available from the British Library

ISBN 0 7225 2774 8

Phototypeset by Harper Phototypesetters Limited,
Northampton, England
Printed in Great Britain by
Mackays of Chatham, Kent

To Frederick with love

Contents

Introduction

Generally, age is measured in chronological terms, but years have very little to do with age in biological terms.

It is difficult to assess accurately age in terms of birthdays, but what is easily recognizable is the visible signs generally associated with advancing years. Ageing skin means a reduction of natural oils, a decrease in cell reproduction, and a loss of elasticity and subcutaneous fat. Such symptoms are usually accompanied by greying, brittle, and thinning hair and muscle wasteage, which results in poor posture.

However, the first age-related changes usually occur prematurely. Johan Bjorksten, the famous age-researcher, suggests that one's potential lifespan is a maximum one hundred and fifty-seven years, and if this is true, then the reason we are falling short of this life expectancy by eighty years and more, is because the cells are degenerating and dying far too quickly.

The ageing process varies from person to person. In some women changes occur fairly early, whereas those who have disciplined themselves to eating wholesome foods, exercising and generally caring for their bodies find that the changes are hardly noticeable at fifty, and may only begin to show in their sixties and seventies, although this is unusual.

Ageing is not one but a combination of factors. Obviously, genetic factors, health and the determination to remain both mentally and physically active and enjoy life are extremely important. So too, is a diet rich in vitamins and minerals, a deficiency of which results in rapid ageing (see pages 39, 52). Stress, smoking, sunbathing regularly, going without a moisturizer and drinking tap water also hasten the ageing process. Less noticeable but equally harmful are the effects of heavy metals and pollutants in the air, found in smog and in industrial and built-up areas. Radiation and environmental pollutants of many kinds collect in the atmosphere and produce toxic, unstable atoms or molecules known as free radicals, which endanger the life of healthy skin cells, impairing the synthesis of proteins and reducing skin elasticity; the result is wrinkled, aged skin. Nevertheless, substances such as the pectin found in apples, oranges and grapefruit remove the heavy metals, while vitamin C combined with vitamin E and other nutrients together kill off free-radicals, and thus protect the skin. Additional protection is possible by applying the Skin Protector Against Free Radicals (see page 109).

All these genetic, health and environmental factors combine to form a lethal cocktail that is likely to damage health and functioning on a cellular level – if you let it! This book provides all the help and encouragement necessary to combat these effects, prevent further signs of ageing and perhaps even 'turn back the clock'. A guide to calories and ideal weight is complemented by a variety of easy-to-follow diets to suit individual needs, with delicious, vitamin-packed recipes. You will find advice on the preparation of simple, homemade beauty preparations such as the Sunflower Hand Cleanser and Honey Under-Eye Treatment, which will improve your appearance and save money too. There are more tips still on how to deal with the special problems that can affect skin, hair, nails, legs and feet. Guidance on practical, safe ways to reduce stress levels and ensure restful sleep without drugs, with advice on exercise, helps you to attain lasting 'ageless beauty' and vitality and *feel* youthful too!

Ageing could be a problem, but it doesn't need to be. So stop worrying and start doing something about it today. You owe it to yourself and your family.

PART ONE

Ageless Vitality from Within

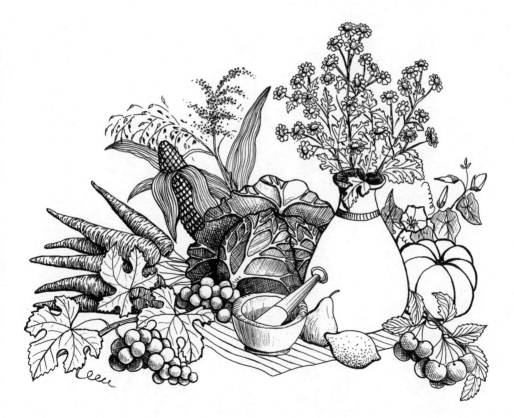

1

Foods for Ageless Beauty

The Wonder Foods and Drinks can transform your diet straightaway, cleansing your system, giving you renewed energy, protecting you against illness and giving you a healthy, youthful glow. These wholesome foods have undergone minimal processing and are bursting with nutritional goodness. Water is also a vital ally in slowing the ageing process: increasing your intake of water eliminates toxins from the body more effectively and ensures proper cell hydration. At the end of this chapter you will find Protein, Vitamin and Mineral Charts, which provide detailed information on function, rich sources, symptoms of deficiency and the Ageless Beauty Dose in each case. These charts are of essential importance and should be studied closely – it is their protein, vitamin and mineral content that gives the Wonder Foods and Drinks their seemingly miraculous powers!

THE WONDER FOODS

Blackstrap Molasses

A by-product of sugar-refining, blackstrap molasses supplies calcium, iron, sodium, copper, phosphorus, potassium, and all the B vitamins including inositol, a lack of which may cause constipation, eczema, abnormalities of the eyes, premature baldness and greying hair. Moreover, it contains more calcium and iron than milk and liver and is an excellent food for women a) suffering from anaemia and fatigue, b) during the menopause when the lack of ovarian hormones causes severe calcium deficiency and c) when lack of nutrients, not advanced years, is indirectly responsible for osteoporosis and brittle bones. Blackstrap molasses has also been used successfully in preventing and alleviating arthritis. It is a marvellous nightcap for those who have difficulty sleeping. Not surprisingly, it is an excellent beautifier too, which with its gentle laxative effect cleanses the system of impurities while nourishing it, thus resulting in clear, unblemished skin and healthy hair.

The finest blackstrap molasses is the unsulphured kind made from the thick residue left over from making sugar out of the sugar cane. Sulphured molasses is bleached to make it more marketable, but during the process important nutrients are destroyed. A general misconception is that black treacle is a synonym for molasses, but the former is much richer in sugar than the type of molasses recommended here.

This wonder food can be substituted for sugar or honey in muffins, cakes, biscuits and other recipes. Alternatively, one teaspoonful of it dissolved in half a cup each of hot water and milk transforms an iron-deficient drink into an iron-rich one.

Brewer's Yeast

Formerly only used in the brewing industry, hence its name, but now produced and sold specifically as a health food supplement, brewer's yeast contains seventeen vitamins including the B complex group, fourteen minerals and sixteen amino acids. In addition, it is a good source of protein, supplying 50 grams of complete protein per half cup compared with 20 grams per half cup of cottage cheese and about 16 grams per half cup of powdered skimmed milk (instant). This wonderful food must not be confused with either fresh yeast or dried baker's yeast, which are leavening agents used in baking.

Evidence suggests that brewer's yeast taken daily acts as a protection against cancer of the liver, helps re-build diseased tissue, strengthens heart muscles and improves circulation. I also recommend it to those who are suffering from acne, dry skin and hair problems and include it in a number of external beauty treatments.

Brewer's yeast is available in both tablet and powder form, but the former is more expensive and it has been estimated that about twenty tablets are needed to satisfy the recommended dose of one tablespoonful daily.

People with adequate diets taking brewer's yeast for the first time may experience indigestion and a 'gassy', full feeling caused by a deficiency of hydrochloric acid, necessary to digest yeast, but persevere. Start by taking a half teaspoonful or less to begin with, and increase the dosage gradually to the full tablespoonful.

To ensure your complement of these nutrients, sprinkle brewer's yeast over wholegrain breakfast cereal or stir it into a glass of milk or fruit juice. I take brewer's yeast in fortified milk in which various nutrients are combined together to achieve maximum absorption. This drink consists of brewer's yeast, semi-skimmed milk, powdered skimmed milk, blackstrap molasses, wheatgerm, vegetable oil, and additional ingredients as and when needed.

Fish and Fish-Oil Concentrates

For centuries, cod-liver oil has been taken as a preventive-cum-cure for a diversity of complaints from bronchitis to rickets, rheumatism and skin disorders, but it was not until 1912 when vitamins were discovered that its function was more fully understood.

Research showed that it was one of the richest sources of vitamins A and D needed for eyes, skin, teeth and gums and for the absorption of calcium and phosphorus so essential for healthy bones, teeth and nails.

The next major advance in the understanding of fish and its properties occurred twenty years ago when Dr Hugh Sinclair, a world authority on nutrition, studying the diet of the Greenland Eskimos, discovered that the death rate from heart disease was only one-eighth that of the USA. Incidences of asthma, diabetes, psoriasis and rheumatoid arthritis were also low compared with those of the West. It was soon discovered that a polyunsaturated fat called eicosapentaenoic acid (EPA), one of three fatty acids in fish, can lower blood fats and prevent blood cells from clotting, thus an EPA-rich diet can reduce the risk of heart attacks.

Trials using cod-liver oil on arthritis sufferers showed noticeable reductions in the symptoms of swollen, tender joints, pain and stiffness. Skin and hair problems, eczema, acne and psoriasis in particular have also been relieved by taking fish oil in the diet.

An excessive level of vitamin D leading to toxicity is rare and can be prevented by taking large quantities of vitamin C, E, and choline, but the fear was such that the National Research Council recommended only 400 international units (two teaspoonfuls) daily, despite individual variations in requirements. Studies undertaken by Dr Johnston of the Henry Ford Hospital in Detroit indicated that adolescents and adults, especially during pregancy and menopause, may benefit from taking approximately 4,000 international units of vitamin D daily.

Steaming, poaching and grilling are good ways of cooking fish.

Add cod-liver oil to milk, shake thoroughly and drink.

Breathe through your mouth and you won't even notice the taste! Fish-oil concentrates are available in capsule form.

Anchovies	High in EPA in spring, lower in winter
Cod-Liver Oil	High in EPA and vitamins A and D
Haddock	Low in EPA. High in phosphorus and potassium
Halibut	Flesh is low in EPA, but liver is high. Also fairly high in vitamin B_3 and potassium
Halibut-Liver Oil	High in EPA and vitamins A and D
Herring	High in EPA and cholesterol and fairly high in vitamins B_2, B_3, B_6, B_{12} and D, as well as phosphorus, calcium and potassium
Kippers	High in EPA. Fairly high in calcium and phosphorus
Lobster	High in EPA and vitamin A, but also high in cholesterol
Mackerel	High in EPA and cholesterol. Fairly high in vitamins B_2, B_3, and phosphorus and potassium
Pilchards	High in EPA
Prawns	High in EPA
Salmon	Medium in EPA, high in cholesterol and fairly high in vitamins B_3, B_{12} and D, and phosphorus and potassium
Sardines	High in EPA. Fairly high in vitamins B_2, B_3, B_{12}, folic acid and D, and all the minerals
Tuna	High in EPA and fairly high in vitamins B_6 and B_{12}
Whitebait	High in EPA

Note The above list is only an approximate guide, for levels vary from season to season.

Fortified Milk

A super food in liquid form, rich in high-quality protein, calcium, phosphorus, potassium and sodium, low in calories and practically free from fat, is fortified milk. The basic ingredients are 4oz (100 grams) powdered skimmed milk (non-instant), and two pints (1.16 litres) of skimmed or semi-skimmed milk, blended together. The result is a creamy-tasting drink that can be added to cereals and beverages and used in cooking.

A number of other health-promoting ingredients can also be added to the above: between one teaspoon and four tablespoons of powdered brewer's yeast (depending on whether or not one is used to yeast, see page 14); one tablespoon of blackstrap molasses;

one tablespoon of lecithin; one teaspoon of calcium lactate; two tablespoons of wheatgerm and one tablespoon of vegetable oil (cold pressed), produces a liquid food that supplies most of the essential nutrients, including all the B vitamins. This sustaining drink should be sipped slowly between meals throughout the day and before going to bed.

Garlic (Vegetable Penicillin)

Whether you love or hate it, garlic with its high sulphur, potassium and phosphorus content is a powerful germicide, antiseptic and cleanser that protects against bacterial and viral infections, cleanses the system of impurities and detoxifies harmful substances which can damage the cells and hasten ageing. Research shows that it lowers cholesterol, which helps to prevent arteriosclerosis, aids digestion and banishes bad breath. Pimples vanish when rubbed several times with garlic.

Garlic-lovers like myself use it at every opportunity to season dishes of all kinds, and the salad bowl rubbed with a clove imparts a lovely tang to salads. Of course, not everyone likes the taste or the smell for that matter, and those who don't can buy capsules of garlic oil that are both tasteless and odourless from health food shops. If one's only concern is its anti-social odour, it can be counteracted by chewing a sprig of parsley or drinking a glass of milk after eating it.

Lecithin

Derived from the Greek word 'likithos' meaning the 'egg of the yolk', lecithin, made up of fat, choline, inositol and unsaturated fatty acids, is a natural substance produced by the liver when the diet is adequate, which breaks down cholesterol deposits on arterial walls into particles so minute that they can be absorbed into the tissues, thus averting coronary disease. It also enables the assimilation of vitamins A, D, E and K.

When an undersupply of lecithin occurs, cholesterol adheres to the inner walls of the arteries and builds up, thus restricting the passage of blood which, if left unchecked, may and often does prove fatal.

Physicians often recommend diets which either restrict or contain no eggs, liver, full milk, butter and other fats high in cholesterol, but foods containing cholesterol are the very ones that also contain lecithin. Only when intakes of choline are low and the production of lecithin adversely affected can these foods increase the cholesterol in the blood. Surely the solution is not to deprive the body of these cholesterol foods, which are necessary for sound nerves and healthy blood cells, but to reduce the intake of processed foods which are low or totally devoid of lecithin and to eat more egg yolk, milk, liver, heart, kidneys, brains, soya beans, sunflower seeds, nuts, vegetable oils (cold pressed), yeast and wheatgerm, which are good sources of lecithin.

Lecithin in granular form (capsules contain too little to be effective), extracted from dried soya beans and taken daily by sprinkling two teaspoonfuls of it over muesli or salads, or adding to yogurt or fortified milk, helps to maintain a healthy heart and nervous system, good eyesight and beautiful skin and hair.

Another pleasant way of taking lecithin is to make soya bean cream.

Soya Bean Cream

1 pint (570ml) soya bean milk
½ pint (285ml) soya bean oil
honey (optional)

Place the milk in a basin, and pour the oil in a continuous trickle, beating continuously until the right consistency is achieved. If the thickness similar to single cream is desired use less oil; for double or thicker cream, use more. Add honey if desired.

Cream, even the ersatz, lecithin-rich kind is unlikely to be taken as often as one would like, but one way of taking it daily is in the form of soya bean butter.

Soya Bean Butter

1 tablespoon soya bean flour
½ pint (285ml) soya bean oil
¼ pint (140ml) water

Mix the water and the flour together. Put in a saucepan, bring to the boil and simmer until it thickens. Strain into a basin, and add the oil a little at a time, beating continuously into a smooth spread. Use instead of ordinary butter on bread.

Liver

Raw liver may not look particularly appetising to the squeamish, but when cooked properly, and this means very lightly, it is quite delicious. Only overcooked liver that is leathery is unpalatable. It is important to try to learn to like liver, for few foods provide such a valuable source of nutrients so cheaply. A treasure-trove of complete protein and minerals including iron, liver also contains appreciable amounts of vitamins A, B_1, B_2, B_6, B_{12}, C and D.

The nutrients in liver help to protect us against toxic substances such as poisoning from chemical insecticides; indeed, doctors trained and interested in human nutrition prescribe it as a dietary supplement to patients suffering from insecticide poisoning. Being rich in iron, it is also effective in treating pernicious anaemia and eliminating fatigue. It also reduces stress and repairs damaged cells, which is vital if one is to remain healthy and youthful.

Experiments carried out at the Sloan Kettering Institute for Cancer Research in New York showed that rats fed desiccated liver in large quantities became immune to artificially induced cancers, whereas other rats similarly treated but deprived of liver died within a matter of days.

Studying Dr Frederick Steigmann's treatment of patients suffering from serious liver disease in the USA, in which crude liver extract and other nutritional improvements were made to the diets, shows a reduction in the death rate by two-thirds. Mr Paul de Kruif in 'Your Liver is Your Life' (*Reader's Digest*, January 1958) commented 'If the nutritional treatment of advanced cirrhosis is so powerfully curative, why not use it to guard the liver while its cells are still normal? If we give our liver the right nutriments to work with, its cells will help to guard themselves. The nutritional supplements added to a good diet can do much like those used in the treatment of a sick liver, but less intensive and expensive.'

Liver's achievements internally are obviously reflected externally in the way we feel and look. Certainly, for clear skin and healthy hair, there is no better beautifier.

This super-food cannot be rated too highly or eaten too frequently. One way of ensuring a regular intake is in the form of desiccated liver made from liver dried at low temperatures to retain its therapeutic properties. It is available in powder or tablet form.

The most amusing tale concerning liver that I have ever heard appeared in Adelle Davis' *Let's Eat Right to Keep Fit*. It concerned a young man who was completing his doctorate at the University of California and suffering from fatigue. Miss Davis prescribed that he should eat ½lb of liver daily for breakfast, but due to a misprint it was mistaken for 2lb of liver each morning. He persisted as best he could, but later she received the following doggerel:

My dear Adelle it is plain hell to follow your directions;
But I do try hard, avoid all lard and all the fine confections.

There is much to encourage and much to intrigue,
So much to be grateful for this lack of fatigue.

With devotion to you and in spite of my pride . . .
One thing that I can hardly abide

Is rising each morning at the clang of clocks
and facing the white vastness of the icebox.
I withdraw with fright and begin to shiver
on seeing that mountain of slippery liver.

But once it is down, I lift high my cup,
And I can drink deep of the milk and pep-up.

Rose-Hips

As any gardener knows, rose-hips are the attractive reddish-orange berries that appear on the boughs of the *Rosa canina* (dog rose), the *R. rugosa* and the *R. rubiginosa* (sweetbriar) after flowering in late autumn and early winter.

During the Second World War when shortages of fresh fruits resulted in a severe vitamin C deficiency in young children, nutritionists discovered that rose-hips were four times as rich in vitamin C as blackcurrants, twenty times as rich as oranges and sixty times as rich as lemons. As a result of their findings, hundreds of tons were harvested to make rose-hip syrup. Even today, this red, sticky liquid is still produced commercially. Synthetic vitamin C, known as ascorbic acid, has its uses, but it is not comparable, nutritionally speaking, to the natural vitamin C found in fresh fruits.

As well as being a powerhouse of vitamin C, rose-hips contain vitamins A, B_1, B_2, E, K and P, together with iron, calcium, and phosphates. When infused, the hips make a herbal tea which acts as a diuretic and so helps to maintain healthy kidneys. Naturally, this tea also aids those wishing to lose weight. In addition, rose-hips may be made into purees, soups, marmalades and jams. Few people have the time, the patience, or the inclination to make rose-hip syrup of their own, but those who would like to try will find it well worth the effort.

Rose-Hip Syrup

1lb (450g) rose-hips
4½ pints (2.5 litres) water (hot, but not boiling)
1¼lb (550g) sugar

Wash the rose-hips thoroughly in cold water, 'top' and 'tail', and mince them in a coarse kitchen mincer. Put the pulpy fruit into either an enamel or a stainless steel saucepan (don't use an aluminium pan which destroys vitamin C and discolours the fruit), add 3 pints (1.7 litres) of hot water, cover, and bring to the boil. After fifteen minutes, remove the pan from the heat and carefully pour the contents through either a clean nylon stocking or a fine flannel bag, so that the liquid filters slowly into a clean basin placed below. When it has drained into the bowl, pour it back into the saucepan, add 1½ pints (850ml) of hot water, stir and leave to stand for a further fifteen minutes. Repeat the straining process at least twice more until there are no fine hairs in the liquid, for if left, they can irritate the stomach. After the final straining, pour the liquid into another clean, enamel or stainless steel saucepan, place it over a low heat, and allow to simmer gently until the quantity of liquid is reduced by half. Finally, add the sugar, boil for a further five minutes, and then pour the syrup into clean bottles. Seal and store in a cool dark place.

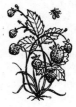

Rose-Hip Tea

Wash, 'top' and 'tail' the fruits and soak them in water overnight. Twelve hours later, drain and put them in an enamel or a stainless steel saucepan, add all the water, cover and place on a low heat to simmer for thirty-five to forty minutes. Then, remove from the heat and when the tea is cool enough to drink, pour yourself a glassful and add honey if desired. This herbal tea is a delicious and simple way of protecting yourself against colds during the winter.

3 tablespoons rose-hips
3 pints (1.7 litres) water (hot but not boiling)
honey (optional)

Rose-Hip Puree

Wash and trim the fruits as before. Pour the water over them, cover, bring to the boil, and leave to simmer for twenty minutes or so, until the hips are quite tender. Press and strain through a fine sieve using a wooden spoon and repeat the filtering process twice more as described in the syrup recipe. The result is a delicious purée for garnishing fish, fowl, or a variety of meat and pasta dishes. Fortify milk and fruit drinks with one tablespoonful of this vitamin C-rich extract.

2lbs (1kg) rose-hips
2 pints (1.15 litres) water

Seeds

Seeds are the embryo of life, packed with concentrated nourishment to produce and sustain new life. People have eaten seeds since the very earliest times: in Genesis, Chapter 1, verse 29, 'God said, "Behold, I have given you every herb bearing seed, which is upon the face of all the earth, and every tree in which is the fruit of a tree yielding seed; to you it shall be for meat." '

Indeed like meat, seeds are high in protein and contain many amino acids, but as with many foods of seed, fruit or vegetable origin, they lack some of the essential amino acids needed by the body to build bones, blood, hair and other protein requirements, the complement only being obtained when they are combined with pulse, cheese or grain dishes. In addition to the amino acids which make up proteins, seeds are an excellent source of vitamins and minerals, and some even contain hormones.

Fat-soluble vitamin A, essential in aiding resistance to infection and maintaining healthy eyes, skin, tooth enamel and mucous membranes, is present in many seeds. The way seeds encapsulate goodness enables the B vitamins in which they are rich to remain fresher and more potent longer than those found in fresh vegetables. Stored in the essential fatty acid within the seed is a good source of vitamin E, a deficiency of which causes anaemia and premature ageing.

Generally, foods such as fruits and vegetables that are high in vitamins are low in phosphorus. Seeds, however, contain this mineral in appreciable quantities, thus enabling the body to utilize the calcium for healthy bones and teeth and for the digestion of protein. Other minerals present in seeds are potassium, magnesium, iron and zinc.

Sunflower Seeds

In Czarist Russia, soldiers were allocated a so-called iron ration which consisted solely of sunflower seeds. More than forty years later, the United States Department of Agriculture rated the protein content of sunflower seeds higher than all other vegetable seeds, and almost as high as steak, which is recommendation indeed from a nation that consumes steaks in such vast quantities!

Once described as 'a little sunlamp in your digestive system', these sun-drenched seeds eaten daily are found to benefit eyesight by both improving vision and acting as a screen against the sun's glare. Further claims include easing arthritis, constipation and reducing high blood pressure and circulatory problems.

'Snacking' on sunflower seeds has the calming effect of nicotine without the addiction or the dangers of smoking, because they contain B vitamins, calcium and essential oils that have a sedative effect.

Sunflower seeds can be added to muesli and breakfast mixtures containing grains and dried fruits. Sunflower, sesame and pumpkin seeds in equal portions, ground in a blender, make a complete protein to sprinkle on soups (just before serving), cereals, yogurts and desserts.

Sunflower Puree

Place the ingredients in a liquidizer and blend until smooth. This nutritious puree, with its lovely nutty flavour, can be added to plain milk or fresh fruit milk shakes.

2oz (50 grams) sunflower seeds (washed)
1 pint (570ml) water

Sesame Seeds

Regarded as a symbol of immortality, sesame was one of the earliest seeds to be cultivated by Man. In the Middle East, sesame seeds ground into a creamy spread called tahini, is an essential part of the staple diet. Like sunflower seeds, sesame seeds are high in protein, oil, vitamins and minerals, but more important still, they are a treasure trove of calcium. One half cup of sesame seeds contains 580mg of calcium whereas the same quantity of milk (whole) contains only 285mg, and sunflower seeds a mere 60mg. Particularly interesting is their high lecithin content, which helps to break down fat and potentially harmful cholesterol deposits on arterial walls.

Either plain, toasted, or sprouted, sesame seeds make satisfying between-meal snacks, and are always included in my tossed salads. Mix with fresh fruits and honey for a healthy dessert.

Sesame Milk

Place all the ingredients in a liquidizer and blend until smooth. This creamy drink, with its slight almond flavour, is delicious!

2oz (50 grams) sesame seeds (washed)
½ pint (285ml) water
½ pint (285ml) milk
1 teaspoon honey

Pumpkin Seeds

Pumpkin seeds are to the Hungarians, Bulgarians and Ukranians, what sunflower seeds are to the Russians; a ready source of Nature's nutrients. These people also know that pumpkin seeds help preserve the prostate gland and thus male potency. Research carried out by Dr W. Devrient of Berlin confirmed that these seeds contain a plant hormone which has a regenerative, invigorative and vitalizing influence on male hormone production. Pumpkin seeds are similar in composition to sunflower and sesame seeds but richer in iron and zinc.

Sprinkle them either whole, ground or sprouted on snacks, muesli, desserts, salads and grain and vegetable dishes.

Wheatgerm

Wheatgerm is a health-cum-beauty food *par excellence* that I am never without. What makes it so special is that unlike wheatbran or wheatflakes, wheatgerm is the life-giving embryo of the wheat, which is rich in all the B vitamins, vitamin E, iron, magnesium, copper, manganese, calcium and phosphorus. Furthermore, it is a good and inexpensive source of complete proteins, containing the eight essential amino acids necessary to sustain life. Wheatgerm contains more protein per half cup than ¼lb of either lean meat, fish, or fowl, and four times more than is found in one egg, and at a fraction of the cost.

These nutrients contained in wheatgerm are believed to rejuvenate and help re-build skin tissue, to heal unsightly scars and to combat fatigue and anaemia, but it is also a remarkable beauty food for curing acne and skin blemishes and promoting strong, healthy hair.

My faith in wheatgerm was confirmed after the sudden death of a close relative twenty years ago. The shock was such that my hair, always long and luxuriant, became so badly matted that the tangled masses had to be cut out, until all that remained were a few shortened, wispy strands. To help re-build my health and my hair, wheatgerm was included in my daily diet and the effect was remarkable. Within three months, the condition of my hair had improved beyond belief, and after just six months, it had thickened up and grown nearly five inches compared with the average rate of nearer three inches.

Raw wheatgerm bought fresh in vacuum packs is the best. Not only is it better for you but far cheaper than the processed kind. Like all worthwhile, fresh foods, it should be refrigerated to keep it 'sweet' and in peak condition.

This tasty and nutritionally rich food can be sprinkled over salads and desserts and added to mueslis and soups, stews and casseroles just before serving. With an electric blender, one can make delicious and fortifying drinks with one pint of either milk or fruit juice, half a cup of wheatgerm, a banana or a few strawberries or similar fruit. Superb muffins, cakes, and breads can be made by substituting between 2 and 4oz (50 and 100 grams) of wheatgerm for an equivalent amount of flour in the recipe.

Yogurt

A fermented milk product cultured by bacteria to produce lactic acid, yogurt aids the absorption of iron and calcium, and supplies vitamins B_2, B_3 in generous quantities together with other vitamins and protein in a form that is easily absorbed. The healthy bacteria in yogurt controls the putrefying bacteria in the intestinal tract and so helps to keep it clean. Real yogurt, known as the 'milk of eternal life', is believed to be the secret of the Bulgarians' youthfulness and longevity, even when extremely advanced in years.

A delicious yogurt, and a favourite of mine, contains no artificial sugar and costs far less than commercial brands. The recipe is as follows:

Homemade Yogurt

Using either a liquidizer or a wooden spoon, blend all the ingredients together until the mixture is smooth. Pour into jars and place either in a yogurt-maker or in a large pan of warm water, which reaches the top of the jars, and leave to simmer over a low heat. Alternatively, a bowl of the mixture can be placed on top of a gas boiler where there is a constant temperature of between 105 and 110°F (c. 40°C). Leave it there for four hours or until it is the consistency of custard. It will need a longer setting time if the temperature drops.

Yogurt can be added to soups immediately prior to serving (cooking kills the beneficial bacteria), or used in salad dressings or on jacket potatoes, or with fresh fruit, or simply eaten by itself.

½lb (225 grams) powdered, skimmed milk
1 large can evaporated milk
2 pints (1.15 litres) water
3 tablespoons yogurt (either a commercial yogurt or the remains of the previous home-made one)

THE WONDER DRINKS
Fruit and Vegetable Juices

Fruit and vegetable juices are shown to possess remarkable healing and health-promoting properties. It is still not fully understood, according to the orthodox study of nutrition, exactly why drinking raw juices has successfully relieved and/or treated hypertension, kidney, heart and blood diseases, rheumatism, diabetes, peptic ulcers, colitis, and intestinal, skin and eye disorders. Raw juices are also believed to help retard ageing and are recommended by nutritionally minded specialists in the prevention of cancers.

Fresh, raw juices contain vital enzymes, which together with vitamins, minerals and trace elements are absorbed and assimilated rapidly in quantities that would otherwise be impractical.

If you are sceptical about juices and their health-giving qualities, consider the case of Dr Norman W. Walker, an early exponent of this principle, who studied the subject for more than fifty years and wrote:

'Every plant, vegetable, fruit, nut and seed in its raw natural state is composed of atoms and molecules. Within these atoms and molecules reside the vital elements we know as enzymes. Enzymes are not things or substances! They are the life principle in the atoms and molecules of every living cell.

'The enzymes in the cells of the human body are exactly like those in vegetation, and the atoms in the human body each have a corresponding affinity for like atoms in vegetation. Consequently, when certain atoms are needed to rebuild or replace body cells, there will come into play a magnetic-like attraction which will draw to such cells in our bodies the exact kind and type of atomic elements from the raw foods we eat.

'Accordingly, every cell in the structure of our bodies and every cell in nature's foods are infused and animated with the silent life known as enzymes. This magnetic-like attraction, however, is only available in live molecules! Enzymes are sensitive to all heat above 130 deg. F. At 130 deg. F they are dead. Any food which has been cooked at a temperature higher than 130 deg. F has been subjected to the death sentence of its enzymes, and is nothing but dead food.

'Naturally, dead matter cannot do the work of live organisms. Consequently, food which has been subjected to higher temperatures above 130 deg. F has lost its live, nutritional value. While such food can, and does, sustain life in the human system, it does so at the expense of progressively degenerating health, energy and vitality'.

Dr Walker, who suffered from neuritis (inflammation of the nerves), a condition which is extremely painful, cured himself by drinking fresh, raw juices and foods every day. He lived a long and active life and died, free of pain and disease, aged 109 in 1986. Such a long and active life is surely proof enough of the miracle of raw juices.

Always select only the freshest and youngest fruits and vegetables for juicing. To capture all the nutrients, wash or scrub under cold, running water, slice, place in a liquidizer, cover with water, blend and drink the juice slowly as soon as it is made. Experiment with different combinations to find the ones that are both to your liking and your requirements. It really is great fun!

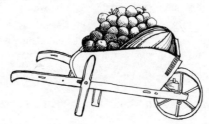

Vegetable Juices

Beetroot

A good, red blood cell builder that improves blood quality and is recommended in cases of anaemia. It is also an excellent cleanser, particularly of the liver and kidneys. Young, unpeeled beetroot liquidized makes a lovely, rich, wine-coloured juice, but its flavour is far from pleasant and it must be added, in small quantities, to other vegetable and fruit juices.

Good Combinations:
1 part beetroot and 2 parts carrot
2 parts beetroot, 8 parts carrot and 3 parts cucumber
1 part beetroot and 2 parts pineapple

Cabbage

A light green juice with a fairly strong flavour that tastes better when combined with other vegetable juices. It cleanses the intestinal tract, is effective in treating constipation and stomach ulcers, and if sipped before meals, is a good way of regulating the appetite. Contains vitamins B_1, B_3, folic acid, C and potassium in high quantities.

Good Combinations:
3 parts cabbage and 2 parts carrot
3 parts cabbage and 1 part tomato
2 parts cabbage, 4 parts carrot and 2 parts lettuce

Carrot

Particularly rich in vitamins A, B_3, folic acid, E, potassium and other vitamins, minerals and trace elements, carrot juice has been used to treat a wide range of disorders from skin, eye and digestive problems to ulcers and even cancerous growths because of the way it both soothes and fights infection.

This juice can be enjoyed by itself, but generally is used as the basic ingredient of juice combinations.

Good Combinations:
1 part carrot and 4 parts orange
2 parts carrot, 1 part lettuce, 1 part turnip and 1 part beetroot
2 parts carrot and 1 part beetroot

2 parts carrot and 3 parts cabbage
1 part carrot, 1 part celery and 1 part spinach
4 parts carrot, 2 parts celery and 1 part parsley
5 parts carrot and 3 parts apple
8 parts carrot, 3 parts cucumber and 2 parts beetroot
4 parts carrot, 2 parts cabbage and 2 parts lettuce
1 part carrot, 1 part celery and 1 part apple
2 parts carrot, 4 parts apple and 1 part orange
8 parts carrot, 5 parts celery and 3 parts cucumber

Celery

Celery juice, which contains vitamins A, B_1, B_2, B_6, B_{12}, folic acid, C and E and the minerals phosphorus, calcium, sodium, iron and potassium, helps to maintain the correct balance of body fluids, making it an ideal cocktail for slimmers and those with a tendency to nervousness. It is also a superb internal cleanser for detoxifying the body tissues.

Good Combinations:
1 part celery, 1 part carrot and 1 part spinach
1 part celery and 2 parts carrot
1 part celery, 1 part carrot and 1 part tomato
2 parts celery, 2 parts tomato and 1 part watercress
4 parts celery, 6 parts apple and 1 part parsley
2 parts celery, 4 parts carrot and 1 part parsley
1 part celery, 1 part carrot and 1 part apple
5 parts celery, 8 parts carrot and 3 parts cucumber

Cucumber

Cucumber contains numerous vitamins and minerals, including particularly high levels of vitamin C and folic acid, and its rich potassium content makes it a good blood pressure regulator. It is also a natural diuretic that flushes out the kidneys and for this reason is recommended in reducing and detoxifying diets. Sliced, unpeeled cucumber liquidized tastes rather bland and must be mixed with other vegetables and fruits.

Good Combinations:
3 parts cucumber, 8 parts carrot and 2 parts beetroot
3 parts cucumber, 8 parts carrot and 5 parts celery
3 parts cucumber and 1 part apple

Lettuce

Lettuce of any kind can be added to any vegetable juices to fortify them, but by using Cos lettuce, you will be doubling the A and C vitamin content. In addition to vitamins A and C, lettuce contains other vitamins and minerals including folic acid in abundance. A natural tranquillizer and diuretic which soothes the stomach, calms the nerves and helps slimmers lose weight.

Good Combinations:
1 part lettuce, 2 parts carrot, 1 part beetroot and 1 part turnip
2 parts lettuce, 4 parts carrot and 2 parts cabbage

Parsley

Parsley juice, using both the leaves and the stalks, is a dark green, extremely potent liquid, rich in chlorophyll, vitamins A, B, C, and E and many minerals including iron. It is beneficial in treating eye, urinary and kidney problems and maintaining healthy adrenal and thyroid glands.

Good Combinations:
1 part parsley, 6 parts apple and 4 parts celery
1 part parsley, 4 parts carrot and 2 parts celery

Spinach

This cocktail rich in vitamins A, B_1, B_2, B_3 and C, and minerals phosphorus, calcium, iron, sodium and potassium, speeds up digestion, cleanses the digestive system, eases constipation and soothes and heals the digestive tract including the colon. Unfortunately, the flavour is strong and so should be used with other vegetables that have a sweet and fairly mild flavour.

Good Combinations:
1 part spinach, 1 part celery and 1 part carrot

Tomato

A delicious appetizer that is high in vitamins A, folic acid, C and the mineral potassium.

Good Combinations:
1 part tomato and 3 parts cabbage
1 part tomato, 1 part celery and 1 part carrot
2 parts tomato, 2 parts celery and 1 part watercress

Watercress

Rich in sulphur, iodine, and many vitamins and other minerals, and a powerful cleanser, watercress juice can be fairly bitter and something of an irritant and so it is best combined with other juices to fortify them. It is used to treat anaemia, emphysema and haemorrhoids.

Good Combinations:
1 part watercress, 2 parts celery and 2 parts tomato
1 part watercress and 8 parts pineapple

Fruit Juices

Apple

Fresh apple juice or 'liquid apples' as I call it, made from unpeeled apples, tastes delicious and is a delightful way of taking vitamins and minerals in large quantities. It has long been used in the treatment of gout and rheumatism and more recently cancer. Apples are plentiful all the year round and blend well with other fruit and vegetable juices.

Good Combinations:
3 parts apple and 5 parts carrot
1 part apple, 1 part celery and 1 part carrot
4 parts apple, 2 parts carrot and 1 part orange
6 parts apple, 4 parts celery and 1 part parsley
1 part apple and 3 parts cucumber

Grape

Fresh grape juice contains vitamins A, many of the B group, C and E plus minerals in appreciable quantities. A good juice for reducing, elimination and detoxifying diets.

Good Combination:
1 part grape and 1 part orange

Grapefruit

The pink-fleshed grapefruit is sweeter and contains up to four times more vitamin A than the white-fleshed variety, but all grapefruit juice is a good source of vitamins and minerals, particularly B_3, B_6, folic acid and C. It is a delicious appetizer before meals.

1 part grapefruit and 2 parts orange
1 part grapefruit, 2 parts orange, 1 part tangerine, 1 part red pepper and 1 part sultanas.

Orange

This golden juice contains good quantities of folic acid, C, potassium and other vitamins and minerals. In common with apple, carrot and celery juices, it helps relieve stress, but above all, it should be sipped and enjoyed for its flavour. It is a luxury to which I look forward daily.

Good Combinations:
1 part orange and 1 part carrot
1 part orange, 4 parts apple and 2 parts carrot
2 parts orange and 1 part grapefruit
5 parts orange and 1 part lemon
2 parts orange, 1 part grapefruit, 1 part tangerine, 1 part red pepper and 1 part sultanas
1 part orange and 1 part pineapple
3 parts orange and 1 part pear

Pear

A good source of folic acid and other vitamins and minerals that aids heart activity and promotes the excretion of excess body fluids. Like orange, it tastes delicious by itself.

Good Combination:
1 part pear and 3 parts orange

Pineapple

Pineapple contains bromelin, an efficient digestant that helps to alleviate the heavy feeling after over-eating. In addition to bromelin, fresh pineapple juice contains seven vitamins plus a minimum of five minerals including potassium.

Good Combinations:
8 parts pineapple and 1 part watercress
1 part pineapple and 1 part orange

My favourite combinations of fruit and vegetable juices:

2 parts apple, 2 parts carrot and 1 part celery
1 part apple, 1 part carrot and 1 sprig parsley
2 parts apple, 2 parts carrot and 1 part cucumber
1 part pear, 1 part carrot and 1 part cabbage

Note The flavour of juices can vary enormously, depending on the growing conditions, age, and freshness of the fruits and vegetables. So, like any good cook, I keep tasting and adding, if necessary, until I achieve the consistency and flavour that suits me. A few drops of lemon or orange juice added to vegetable juices help retain colour and improve flavour.

Other Fruit and Vegetable Health Drinks

Carrot Milk Shake

½ pint (285ml) carrot juice
½ pint (285ml) milk

Place the ingredients in a shaker and mix thoroughly.

A lovely rich cocktail of vitamin A, B_1, B_2, B_3, B_6, B_{12}, folic acid, C, D, and E plus phosphorus, calcium, iron, sodium, potassium, magnesium and other minerals. This superior type of milk shake is particularly suitable for those who are ill, infirm or recuperating from an illness.

Apple Molasses Juice

4 eating apples (cored but unpeeled)
3 teaspoons molasses

Place the ingredients in a liquidizer, cover with water, and blend until smooth. This delicious concoction containing vitamins A, B_1, B_2, B_3, B_6, folic acid, C, E, plus phosphorus, calcium, iron, sodium, potassium and magnesium, combined with its slightly laxative effect, is a healthy way to start the day.

Honeyed Pineapple

Place the ingredients in a liquidizer, cover with water, and blend until smooth.

   This refreshing drink containing vitamins A, B₁, B₂, B₃, B₆, folic acid, C, phosphorus, calcium, iron, sodium, potassium and magnesium is delicious any time of the day.

*½ small pineapple
(peeled and sliced)
3 teaspoons honey*

Rhubarb and Strawberry Special

Blend all the ingredients together, with sufficient water, in a liquidizer until smooth. This drink packed with vitamins and minerals acts as a mild laxative and so one glassful per day is quite sufficient.

*1lb (450g) rhubarb
pieces (young)
½lb (225 grams)
strawberries
2 teaspoons black
molasses*

Get Up and Go Drink

Blend all the ingredients together in a liquidizer until smooth. This lovely, frothy drink, which I named Get Up and Go because it makes you do just that, and gives you energy to spare, is packed with first-class protein, vitamins and minerals, and is perfect for those who can't face breakfast.

   Pour half into a tall glass and sip slowly. The remainder can be enjoyed either just before leaving for work or later as a mid-morning 'pick-me-up'.

*1½ pints (850ml)
milk (low fat)
1 banana (ripe)
1 egg (raw)
2 tablespoons
powdered protein
2 tablespoons
wheatgerm flakes
1 tablespoon lecithin
1 tablespoon
brewer's yeast
(powdered)
honey to taste
(optional)*

Fruit Flip

Place the ingredients in a liquidizer and blend until smooth.

*¼ pint (140ml)
carrot juice
¼ pint (140ml)
orange juice
¼ pint (140ml)
water
1 banana
1 tablespoon
wheatgerm flakes
3 dates (stoned)*

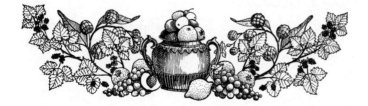

Energy Cup

¾ pint (425ml)
milk (low fat)
¼ pint (140ml)
orange juice
(fresh)
¼ pint (140ml)
carrot juice (fresh)
2 tablespoons yogurt
(plain and
fat-free)
1 tablespoon lecithin
1 tablespoon milk
(dried)
1 teaspoon molasses
(blackstrap)
1 teaspoon honey
(optional)
1 tablespoon
brewer's yeast
(powdered)

Place all the ingredients in a liquidizer and blend until smooth. High in protein, vitamins and minerals, this drink is invaluable when you have a long day ahead of you.

When I need instant energy that has to be sustained for long periods, I begin the day with the Get Up and Go drink and sip the Energy Cup for the remainder of the day. Even if you can't stop to eat, you'll find these health drinks satisfying and very sustaining.

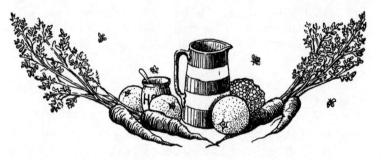

Glamour Girl Sip

½ pint (285ml)
apple juice (fresh)
½ pint (285ml)
carrot juice (fresh)
2 tablespoons yogurt
(plain)
1 teaspoon brewer's
yeast (powdered)
2oz (50 grams)
raisins

Place all the ingredients in a liquidizer and blend until smooth. Containing vitamins A, B_1, B_2, B_6, B_{12}, folic acid, C, E and phosphorus, calcium, iron, sodium, potassium and magnesium, this all-round health drink is particularly helpful to those with spots, pimples, constipation and sluggish livers.

Beauty Cocktail

½ pint (285ml)
strawberry juice
(fresh)
6 dates (stoned)

Place the ingredients in a liquidizer, add a little water and blend until smooth. The resulting fruit cocktail, taken regularly, helps clear spots and other impurities from the complexion.

Golden Glory

Place the ingredients in a liquidizer and blend until smooth.

I enjoy this drink on a hot, summer's day when I don't feel like eating but need an energizer to give me a 'boost'.

½ pint (285ml)
  orange juice
  (fresh)
¼ pint (140ml)
  papaya juice
  (fresh)
1½ teaspoonfuls
  honey (optional)
1 teaspoonful
  brewer's yeast
1 egg

Pineapple Puree

Place the ingredients in a liquidizer and blend until smooth. A good laxative and digestant.

¾ pint (425ml)
  pineapple juice
  (fresh)
¼ pint (140ml)
  prune juice (fresh)
1 tablespoon yogurt
  (plain)
2 teaspoons
  wheatgerm flakes
1 teaspoon lecithin
  powder
1 banana

Health and Beauty Cocktail

½ pint (285ml)
tomato juice
(fresh)
¼ pint (140ml)
carrot juice (fresh)
¼ pint (140ml)
celery juice (fresh)
1oz (25 grams)
parsley (fresh)
1oz (25 grams)
watercress
1 teaspoon lemon
juice
2 tablespoons
wheatgerm flakes
1 tablespoon sesame
oil
1 tablespoon lecithin
powder
2 teaspoons brewer's
yeast (powdered)

Place all the ingredients in a liquidizer and blend until smooth.

This nutritious cocktail is an excellent liquid food. One cup three times a day will help to keep your hair, skin and body glowing with health and vitality.

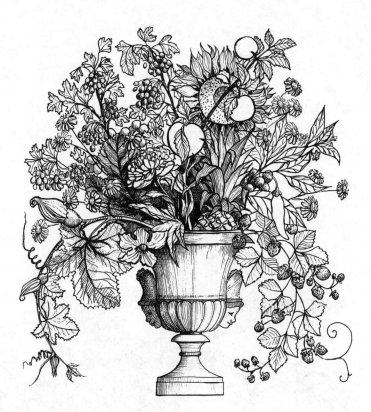

WATER – ARE YOU DRINKING ENOUGH?

Water is vital to life. It is an essential constituent of cells and all body fluids, bathes and purifies blood and tissues, thus cleansing them of poisons and waste matter, and regulates body temperature and body processes. Without it we would die.

However, water in quantities that are sufficient to ensure survival is not necessarily enough to keep us really healthy, least of all actually slow down the ageing process. A lack of moisture over a prolonged period results in slower elimination of toxins that cause loss of vitality, health and premature ageing. It is also known to put a strain on the heart that can actually shorten life. Indeed, this degeneration is slowly happening to most of us now. For the fact is that few of us drink as much water as we should. Even though we are aware of the dangers of dehydration, we are still surprised to see lines and wrinkles appearing relatively early. Yet, this is only the beginning. Internal changes are also occurring. The cells become progressively more dry, and as they dehydrate, so they become less efficient. Calcium, cholesterol, and other substances that normally would be flushed away, remain in the cells, and this is a factor among many that brings about premature ageing. Obviously, cell dehydration is not the sole cause of ageing, but the external effects of stress, smoking, drinking, sun and free-radical damage and other environmental factors might be reduced if cells were kept well watered.

As a result of our civilization and culture, our natural body signals for eating, drinking, sleeping etc. have been repressed and re-scheduled to a routine of our own making. We eat, drink, and sleep at the times specified, rather than when we feel hungry, thirsty and tired. When we feel thirsty, the body is signalling for water of between one and two pints, but we respond by drinking a cup of tea or coffee, or beer, Coca-Cola or some other popular drink that contains diuretics that encourages still more fluids to be excreted from the body. Consequently, instead of being replenished, the tissues become more dry with each passing day.

So how do we know if the tissues are dehydrated? In addition to thirst, the most obvious symptoms are dry skin and lips, constipation, reduced urine, dark-coloured urine, and a dry, grey or coated tongue, the latter perhaps being the most reliable indication of all.

The quantity of water required depends to some extent on the type of foods consumed. Naturally, a person who eats plenty of raw, fresh fruits, vegetables and other foods with a naturally high water content needs less additional liquid than one who lives on starchy, high-carbohydrate foods. Climate too is another factor. Generally however, six to eight glasses or the equivalent of between three and four pints of water daily is recommended for people in temperate climates.

Changing your drinking habits is difficult to begin with but it actually becomes enjoyable as you become accustomed to it. If your intake exceeds the recommended four pints a day, so much the better, for your need for water increases with age. Water taken daily after a lifetime without it won't suddenly reverse the ageing that has already taken place, but it will stop or slow down the process from now on.

PROTEINS AT A GLANCE

Function: Proteins are needed for growth and for the maintenance of the healthy blood cells, tissues, muscles and organs that combine to create a healthy body.

Good Sources	Quantity	Grams of Protein
Steak	¼lb (100 grams)	21
Beef (lean)	¼lb (100 grams)	20
Liver (calf's)	¼lb (100 grams)	21
Chicken	¼lb (100 grams)	23
Turkey	¼lb (100 grams)	22
Fish (average)	¼lb (100 grams)	21
Egg	standard	6
Milk (whole)	½ pint (285ml)	8
Milk (skimmed)	½ pint (285ml)	9
Milk (powdered skimmed, non-instant)	2oz (50 grams)	26
Cheese (cheddar)	2oz (50 grams)	14
Cottage Cheese (uncreamed)	4oz (100 gram)	19
Nuts	2oz (50 grams)	15–22
Soya beans (cooked)	4oz (100 grams)	20
Soya bean flour	2oz (50 grams)	30
Brewer's yeast (powdered)	2oz (50 grams)	50
Desiccated liver	2oz (50 grams)	56
Wheatgerm	2oz (50 grams)	24

Recommended Daily Adult Intake: 46–60 grams

Recommended Daily Child (under 4) Intake: 20–40 grams

Symptoms of Deficiency: General weakness accompanied by little resistance to infection. The hair and nails suffer a check in growth. In extreme cases, patients may suffer loss of hair colour and heart and liver failure.

VITAMINS

Vitamin Weights

1 gamma = 1 microgram (mcg)
1 microgram = 1/1000 of a milligram (mg)
1 milligram = 1/1000 of a gram (gm)
1 gram = 1/30 of an ounce (oz)

VITAMIN CHART

Vitamin A (Retinol)

Function	For healthy skin, eyes, throat, ears, lungs, body tissues, bones, teeth and all bodily repairs. Also helps fight infection and is an important anti-stress vitamin.
Rich sources	Milk (whole, fresh and powdered), butter, margarine, eggs, liver, fish-liver oils, and apricots
Destroyed by	Sunlight and air
Ageless Beauty Daily Adult Dose	15,000–20,000iu
Recommended Daily Adult Dose	5,000iu

Vitamin A (Retinol) continued

Recommended Daily Child Dose	2,000–5,000iu (depending on age)
Symptoms of deficiency	Night blindness and inflammation of the eyes, and dry, flakey, and prematurely ageing skin
Comment	This vitamin, which is needed for all the body's processes, is stored in the liver, and high intakes far in excess of requirements are neither necessary nor advisable. Do not take this vitamin in pill form, for overdosage, though rare, could result in headaches, and loss of hair and appetite

Vitamin B₁ (Thiamine)

Function	For the conversion of carbohydrates into energy. Maintains healthy functioning of the heart, liver, nervous and digestive systems. Helpful in alleviating fatigue and in the treatment of stress, and alcoholism
Rich sources	Milk (fortified), brewer's yeast and blackstrap molasses
Destroyed by	Overcooking, water, air and high temperatures
Ageless Beauty Daily Adult Dose	10–500mg
Recommended Daily Adult Dose	0.9–1.4mg
Recommended Daily Child Dose	0.5–1.4mg (depending on age)
Symptoms of deficiency	Fatigue and poor memory

Vitamin B₂ (Riboflavin)

Function	Needed to metabolize proteins, fats and carbohydrates. Important too, for cell respiration and tissue maintenance, which, as a result, helps prevent premature ageing. Essential for good skin, hair, nails and vision
Rich sources	Fortified milk, lamb's liver, kidney, desiccated liver and brewer's yeast
Destroyed by	Overcooking and over-exposure to light
Ageless Beauty Daily Adult Dose	10–150mg
Recommended Daily Adult Dose	1.2–1.7mg
Recommended Daily Child Dose	0.5–1.4mg (depending on age)
Symptoms of deficiency	Splitting around the mouth, dryness around the nose and on the forehead, oily skin, dandruff, loss of hair and sore eyes that are over-sensitive to light

Vitamin B₃ (Niacin)

Function	Contributes to the breakdown of proteins, fats and carbohydrates and the absorption of cholesterol. Boosts circulation and is essential to the nervous system and to mental health, and for this reason is used to treat mental disorders including schizophrenia. Also necessary for a fine, clear complexion and is used to clear up many skin disorders
Rich sources	Fortified milk, chicken livers, kidney, tuna, wholewheat bread, wheatgerm, sunflower seeds, desiccated liver, brewer's yeast and blackstrap molasses

Destroyed by	Overcooking, so it is believed, but the exact cause is uncertain. Water also destroys some of the vitamin content
Ageless Beauty Daily Adult Dose	100–3,000mg
Recommended Daily Adult Dose	13–19mg
Recommended Daily Child Dose	9–22mg (depending on age)
Symptoms of deficiency	Skin and digestive problems sometimes accompanied by diarrhoea, bad breath, fatigue and nervousness

---

Vitamin B₅ (Pantothenic Acid)

Function	Aids in the function of the adrenal glands and helps combat stress. Also needed for digestion and has been used in therapeutic doses to prevent allergic reactions and digestive upsets and prevent age degeneration
Rich sources	Heart, rice (brown), lentils, peas and brewer's yeast
Destroyed by	Dry heat and acids such as vinegar
Ageless Beauty Daily Adult Dose	50–500mg
Recommended Daily Adult Dose	10–50mg
Recommended Daily Child Dose	2.5–5.0mg (depending on age)

Vitamin B₅ (Pantothenic Acid) continued

Symptoms of deficiency	Irritability, fatigue, nervous headaches, stomach cramps and muscle pains as 'pins and needles'. A deficiency of this vitamin in rats causes premature greying of the hair

Vitamin B₆ (Pyridoxine)

Function	Important in the formation of antibodies, healthy blood cells, and skin tissue and as such, helps to prevent premature skin and hair degeneration. Enables the metabolism to break down proteins, fats and sugars, and is needed for the functioning of the central nervous system and muscle development
Rich sources	Heart, liver, kidney, wheatgerm, wheatbran and blackstrap molasses
Destroyed by	Cooking and oral contraceptives
Ageless Beauty Daily Adult Dose	50–500mg
Recommended Daily Adult Dose	1.6–2.5mg
Recommended Daily Child Dose	0.3–1.2mg (depending on age)
Symptoms of deficiency	Nervousness, irritability, depression, anaemia, eczema, acne and other skin problems, and muscular weakness

Vitamin B₁₂ (Cyanocobalamin)

Function	Essential in the growth of body cells and therefore is linked to ageing and its prevention. Also involved in the

production of red blood cells and in the maintenance of the nervous and reproductive systems

Rich sources   Liver, meat, milk, cheese and eggs

Destroyed by   Heat and cooking in water

Ageless Beauty Daily
* Adult Dose*   50–500mcg

Recommended Daily
* Adult Dose*   3–6mcg

Recommended Daily
* Child Dose*   0.3–2mcg (depending on age)

Symptoms of deficiency   Pernicious anaemia, insomnia, depression and poor concentration and memory

---

Biotin (Vitamin B Complex)

Function   Stimulates cell growth and is involved in the metabolism of food

Rich sources   Brewer's yeast followed by rice bran and germ, wheatbran, nuts, eggs and liver

Destroyed by   Exposure to light. Antibiotics, sulpha drugs and the raw whites of eggs also disrupt its production in the intestines

Ageless Beauty Daily
* Adult Dose*   50–300mcg

Recommended Daily
* Adult Dose*   Not yet determined, but 300mcg appears sufficient

Recommended Daily Child Dose	Not yet determined
Symptoms of deficiency	Anaemia, greyish skin, and depression

Choline (Vitamin B Complex)

Function	Aids distribution of fats from the liver and is needed by the immune system to protect against disease. It is used in the reduction and prevention of high blood pressure and helps restore the natural colour to prematurely grey hair
Rich sources	Pigs liver, legumes, peas, nuts, wholegrains, brewer's yeast and blackstrap molasses
Destroyed by	Alkalis
Ageless Beauty Daily Adult Dose	3,000mg
Recommended Daily Adult Dose	Not yet determined, but estimated to be 3,000–5,000mg
Recommended Daily Child Dose	Not yet determined
Symptoms of deficiency	High blood pressure, haemorrhage of the kidneys, loss of nerve functions, and listlessness. In extreme cases, paralysis and heart attacks may result

Folic Acid (Vitamin B Complex)

Function	Needed in the assimilation of proteins, vitamins A, D, E and K, all of which are oil-soluble and in the formation of red blood cells. It is believed to be important in preventing premature ageing. Also necessary for mental health
Rich sources	Liver, yeast, nuts and green vegetables
Destroyed by	Both cooking and processing for it is sensitive to heat, air and light
Ageless Beauty Daily Adult Dose	800–5,000mcg
Recommended Daily Adult Dose	400–800mcg
Recommended Daily Child Dose	50–300mcg (depending on age)
Symptoms of deficiency	Anaemia, depression, skin and digestive disorders

Inositol (Vitamin B Complex)

Function	Enables the absorption of vitamin E and plays an important role in preventing fatty deposits accumulating in the arteries. It is also needed for healthy hair, brain cells, heart, liver and muscles, and has been used to treat nerve damage resulting from disease, eliminate fatty deposits in the liver and lower cholesterol
Rich sources	Rice, wheatgerm, wholegrains, peas, oranges and grapefruit
Destroyed by	Not yet determined

Inositol (Vitamin B Complex) continued

Ageless Beauty Daily *Adult Dose*	300–800mg
Recommended Daily *Adult Dose*	Not yet determined
Recommended Daily *Child Dose*	Not yet determined
Symptoms of deficiency	Loss of hair, eczema, constipation and high cholesterol levels

PABA (Para-Aminobenzoic Acid – Vitamin B Complex)

Function	Needed for the formation of red blood cells and for maintaining skin and hair health. It has been used to treat skin disorders and with folic acid and pantothenic acid has reversed the greying of hair
Rich sources	Liver, eggs, wheatgerm and blackstrap molasses
Destroyed by	Not yet determined
Ageless Beauty Daily *Adult Dose*	250–500mg
Recommended Daily *Adult Dose*	Not yet determined, but as much as 48,000mg have been given without toxicity
Recommended Daily *Child Dose*	Not yet determined
Symptoms of deficiency	Eczema, fatigue, nervousness, depression, and digestive disorders

Comment	The B vitamins, in the form of brewer's yeast or a B complex formula, taken in excess of bodily requirements are excreted and as such need to be taken daily. Brewer's yeast or B complex tablets need to be well balanced. If the B formula contains 2mg B_1, it should also contain: 2mg B_2 (or equal quantities), 2mg B_6 (or equal quantities), 2mg folic acid (or equal quantities), 20mg pantothenic acid (or ten times the quantity), 20mg niacin (or ten times the quantity), 40mg PABA (or twenty times the quantity), 1,000mg inositol (or five hundred times the quantity), 1,000 mg choline (or five hundred times the quantity), 1–3mg B_{12} (or between half and one-and-a-half times the quantity). Check your formula and see how it compares

Vitamin C (Ascorbic Acid)

Function	Known primarily as the vitamin that fights infection, vitamin C also aids in the formulation of collagen, a protein which protects the cells and gives a certain elasticity to the skin. It also helps prevent coronary heart disease, protects the body against the damage caused by pollutants, poisons and heavy metals, and delays fatigue, thus giving it the reputation of being something of an energiser. It has been used in large doses to treat skin problems and retard the ageing process
Rich sources	Orange juice (fresh), grapefruit, papaya, peppers, watercress, broccoli
Destroyed by	Heat, air, light, prolonged storage, overcooking and iron and copper utensils. Smoking and drugs are responsible for robbing the body of this vitamin

Ageless Beauty Daily
   Adult Dose   80–4,000mg

Recommended Daily
   Adult Dose   60–80mg

Recommended Daily
   Child Dose   40–80mg (depending on age)

Symptoms of deficiency   Susceptibility to infection including gum infection and tooth decay, anaemia, painful joints and weakness of the muscles and bleeding in the nose and mouth

---

Vitamin D (Calciferol)

Function   Essential for the metabolic functions directly concerned with the eyes, heart and nervous system, vitamin D also absorbs calcium and assimilates the sugar and phosphorus necessary for energy and for the development of bones and teeth

Rich sources   Cod, tuna, sardines, salmon, fish-liver oils and butter

Destroyed by   Rancid fats

Ageless Beauty Daily
   Adult Dose   400–1,500iu

Recommended Daily
   Adult Dose   400iu

Recommended Daily
   Child Dose   400iu (depending on age)

Symptoms of deficiency   Brittle bones, hardening of the arteries and in extreme cases, rickets

Comments	Vitamin D, which needs fat for its absorption, is primarily stored in the liver, and therefore quantities in excess of bodily requirements can be toxic, but toxicity can be avoided with generous intakes of C, E and choline

Vitamin E (Tocopherol)

Function	Many wonderful results have been attributed to this vitamin including delaying the effects of premature ageing, healing burns and preventing scarring, treating varicose veins by improving circulation, dispersing blood clots and preventing new ones from forming and alleviating many female problems. Though still something of an enigma, this vitamin is known to protect the cells from damage and the B complex and C vitamins from destruction. It is also needed for the production of new cells, the repair of damaged tissues and has been used in the treatment of scarred skin and damaged livers
Rich sources	Peanuts, wheatgerm, and corn, peanut, olive and safflower oils (cold pressed)
Destroyed by	Cooking, storage, and rancid fats
Ageless Beauty Daily Adult Dose	140–600iu
Recommended Daily Adult Dose	12–15iu
Recommended Daily Child Dose	4–9iu (depending on age)
Symptoms of deficiency	Cancer that is the result of oxygen deficiency in the living cells, fragile red blood cells that rupture easily, prematurely wrinkled and aged skin, and poor muscle tone

Vitamin K

Function	Essential in the production of prothrombin, a protein which is needed for blood coagulation, thus enabling wounds to heal. It also helps to reduce high blood pressure and aids liver functions
Rich sources	Milk, yogurt, eggs, and green, leafy vegetables
Destroyed by	Rancid fats, antibiotics, diarrhoea, colitis, jaundice and any other disorders which hinder or disrupt the production of bile and thus prevent absorption
Ageless Beauty Daily Adult Dose	300–500mcg
Recommended Daily Adult Dose	Not yet determined, but 300–500mcg is considered sufficient
Recommended Daily Child Dose	Not yet determined
Symptoms of deficiency	Haemorrhages
Comment	This vitamin is also produced in intestinal bacteria and provided the diet contains the foods mentioned above, the healthy body is able to produce all that is required

Vitamin P

Vitamin P is one of many complex nutrients that make up bioflavinoids. It occurs naturally wherever vitamin C is present.

Note The Recommended Daily Dose for Adults and Children (RDA) is the UK Recommended Daily Amount believed to be adequate for the nutritional needs of the average individual, while iu stands for international units. However, the nutritional needs of the individual for optimum health and delaying the ageing process varies, but exact dosages have still to be established.

MINERAL AND TRACE ELEMENT CHART
Calcium

Function	Necessary for the formation and the continued maintenance of healthy bones, teeth, tissues, muscles and nerve cells. Also a pain-killer par excellence, which helps alleviate pain, aids blood clotting, which can be a matter of life or death after an accident or serious operation, and hastens recovery. Its tranquillizing effect induces relaxation and untroubled sleep.
Good sources	Milk (powdered, skimmed, or buttermilk), yogurt, cheddar cheese, cottage cheese (homemade), molasses, nuts (unsalted), soya beans, sesame seeds, broccoli, collards, turnip and beet greens, sardines and mackerel.
Concentrates	Bone-meal tablets with vitamin D; calcium tablets; calcium's gluconate and lactate.
Ageless Beauty Daily Adult Dose	1,000–1,500mg
Recommended Daily Adult Dose	800–1,200mg
Recommended Daily Child Dose	800–1,200mg (depending on age)
Symptoms of deficiency	Porous, brittle bones, a susceptibility to tooth decay, and stomach cramps at the onset of menstruation, resulting in nervous tension, irritability and depression
Comments	Calcium is the body's life support, and one of the greatest assets to beauty. A diet high in concentrated carbohydrates, or sweets, or alkaline substances, soda for example, reduces or prevents the absorption of calcium

Chromium

Function	Essential in utilizing sugar and so helps to prevent fatigue. Also believed to be instrumental in keeping cholesterol levels low
Good sources	Brewer's yeast, nuts, fruits and green vegetables
Ageless Beauty Daily Adult Dose	3mg
Recommended Daily Adult Dose	Not defined
Recommended Daily Child Dose	Not defined
Symptoms of deficiency	Laboratory animals lacking chromium develop high or low blood sugar levels, and severe eye abnormalities. In humans, it could also contribute to hardening of the arteries

Copper

Function	Needed for the production of ribonucleic acid (RNA) which is the nucleus of every cell. Aids in the formation of bones, brains, nerves, connective tissue and their functions and helps preserve the natural colour of the hair
Good sources	Liver, kidney and brains
Ageless Beauty Daily Adult Dose	2mg
Recommended Daily Adult Dose	2mg

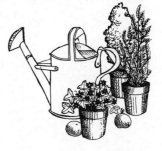

Recommended Daily Child Dose	Not defined
Symptoms of deficiency	The lifespan of red blood cells is shortened, resulting in anaemia. Studies in animals show that skin rashes, hair loss, bone porosity and heart damage resulting in sudden death also occur

Iodine

Function	Essential for the functioning of the thyroid gland that affects growth, physical and mental development and continued good health. Also protects against radioactive fallout
Good sources	Shellfish, sea-fish, kelp, seaweed, sea-salt and other sea foods
Concentrates	Kelp powder; multi-mineral tablets
Ageless Beauty Daily Adult Dose	100–130mcg
Recommended Daily Adult Dose	100–130mcg
Recommended Daily Child Dose	A trace
Symptoms of deficiency	Swelling of the thyroid gland, known as goitre, results in apathy and fatigue, slow pulse, low blood pressure, dry skin, brittle hair and a tendency to gain weight quickly on a low calorie intake. Also associated with a high rate of thyroid cancer, high blood cholesterol, and heart disease

Iron

Function	Vital for the formation of haemoglobin and the transportation of oxygen to the cells. Iron raises the body's energy level and imparts a glow to skin and a lustre to hair
Good sources	Liver, kidney, egg yolk, apricots, brewer's yeast, blackstrap molasses (unsulphured), sesame seeds, soya beans and flour and wheatgerm
Concentrates	Iron tablets; multi-mineral tablets
Ageless Beauty Daily Adult Dose	18–40mg
Recommended Daily Adult Dose	10–18mg
Recommended Daily Child Dose	8–18mg (depending on age)
Symptoms of deficiency	Anaemia, pallid skin, fatigue, loss of energy, dizziness, palpitations, shortness of breath and brittle nails
Comments	'Acidic' foods such as yogurt, buttermilk and citrus fruits and juices aid the absorption of iron. Conversely, carbohydrates interfere with its absorption

Magnesium

Function	Needed by every cell in the body for the absorption and the utilization of proteins, fats and carbohydrates involved in the production of energy. Necessary for muscle and nerve functions. Helps prevent arteriosclerosis by lowering blood cholesterol and is a natural tranquillizer

Good sources	Nuts, soya beans and green, leafy vegetables
Concentrates	Multi-mineral tablets
Ageless Beauty Daily Adult Dose	300–700mg
Recommended Daily Adult Dose	300–350mg
Recommended Daily Child Dose	150–250mg (depending on age)
Symptoms of deficiency	Difficult to detect in humans. Animals lacking magnesium develop convulsions, kidney damage, heart disease and haemorrhages. Conversely, people whose diet is rich in this trace element are found to be free from arteriosclerosis and heart attacks
Comments	A proportionally high intake of magnesium to calcium can inhibit the absorption of the latter. The correct ratio is 1:2 or a minimum daily intake of 300mg of magnesium to 600mg of calcium

Manganese

Function	Activates enzymes and utilizes fats. Has been used to treat heart disease and myasthenia gravis, a chronic muscular disease
Good sources	Nuts, bran, wheatgerm and green, leafy vegetables
Concentrates	Multi-mineral tablets
Ageless Beauty Daily Adult Dose	5–35mg

Recommended Daily Adult Dose	Not defined, but believed to be between 2.5 and 5mg
Recommended Daily Child Dose	Not defined
Symptoms of deficiency	Animals show signs of retarded development, abnormal bone and joint deformities, bad co-ordination, sterility, and loss of sexual drive
Comments	A diet high in phosphorus reduces the absorption of this trace element

Phosphorus

Function	Phosphorus, calcium and vitamin D combine together to build and maintain teeth and skeletal structure. Phosphorus also regulates the chemical balance of the cells, assures mental alertness, hastens muscular response and calms nerves. As the sea at night glows with phosphorescent light, so the skin has a radiance associated with a healthy lifestyle.
Good sources	Fish, meat (lean), poultry, egg yolk, cottage cheese (homemade), milk, powdered milk, yogurt, whole grains, soya beans and nuts
Concentrates	Multi-mineral supplement with vitamin D; bone-meal
Ageless Beauty Daily Adult Dose	800–1,000mg
Recommended Daily Adult Dose	800–1,000mg
Recommended Daily Child Dose	800mg (depending on age)

Symptoms of deficiency	Phosphorus is available in many foods and so there is little danger of a deficiency

Potassium

Function	Controls sodium and so helps to maintain a balance of fluids. Regulates heart beat and muscle control
Good sources	Meat, fruits, vegetables, nuts and wholegrains
Concentrates	Multi-mineral tablets
Ageless Beauty Daily Adult Dose	Approximately 100mg depending on salt intake
Recommended Daily Adult Dose	Not defined, but 5,000mg daily is needed for each teaspoonful of salt consumed
Symptoms of deficiency	Listlessness, fatigue, constipation, insomnia, slow, weak pulse, low blood sugar and general degeneration of the heart
Comments	A balance between potassium and sodium is important: a diet high in one results in a loss of the other

Selenium

Function	Combats environmental toxins such as radiation, helps the immune system to detoxify mercury, lead, cadmium and other heavy metals, and protects against malignancies
Good sources	Tuna, shellfish, kidney, liver, garlic, mushrooms and Canadian wheat

Concentrates	Organic selenium tablets, especially those containing L-selenomethionine, a form of selenium found in foods
Ageless Beauty Daily Adult Dose	70mcg
Recommended Daily Adult Dose	Not defined, but 70mcg is recommended by the Academy of Sciences in the USA
Symptoms of deficiency	Indications are that it can cause cancer and heart disease
Comments	Arthritis has been relieved by taking selenium in tablet form as a regular dietary supplement

Sodium

Function	Works in partnership with potassium to maintain fluid balance, acid-alkali levels and healthy nervous and muscular systems and all cellular metabolism
Good sources	Seafood, cheese, bacon, peanut butter, prepared foods and table salt
Ageless Beauty Daily Adult Dose	None
Recommended Daily Adult Dose	3–7 grams, but now it is believed to be 1 gram or less
Symptoms of deficiency	Headaches, nausea, diarrhoea, muscular cramps and weariness and fatigue in hot weather, extreme cases resulting in exhaustion and heatstroke

Sulphur

Function	Aids in the formation of body tissue and resists bacterial infection. Known as the 'beauty mineral', it is associated with clear skin, shining hair and strong nails and contributes to the body's health and beauty
Good sources	Fish, poultry, eggs, cheese and wheatgerm
Ageless Beauty Daily Adult Dose	10–20mg
Recommended Daily Adult Dose	Not determined, but more than adequate amounts are available in protein foods
Recommended Daily Child Dose	As above
Symptoms of deficiency	Usually those associated with a protein deficiency

Zinc

Function	Helps in the action of enzymes, the formation of proteins and the re-building of cells
Good source	Shellfish
Concentrates	Multi-mineral tablets
Ageless Beauty Daily Adult Dose	15–600mg
Recommended Daily Adult Dose	15–20mg

Recommended Daily Child Dose	3–10mg (depending on age)
Symptoms of deficiency	Poor resistance to infection, slow healing, retarded growth and skin infections. Indications are that deficiencies are common in the West
Comments	A diet high in phosphorus can result in a zinc deficiency

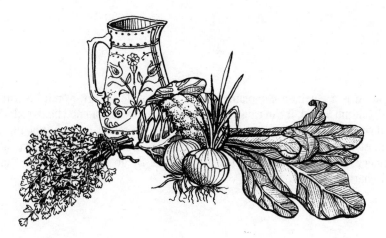

2
Constipation

Constipation is a common complaint that is responsible for an overall deterioration of health. If left untreated, it can cause lethargy, varicose veins, haemorrhoids (piles), cancer of the bowel and diseases which result from the systematic poisoning of the organs.

The most common cause is a lack of roughage in the diet. Other dietary factors are a deficiency of inositol, choline, niacin, vitamin B_1 or potassium (see vitamin and mineral charts pages 39, 52).

NATURAL LAXATIVE FOODS
Blackstrap Molasses

Blackstrap molasses, with its high inositol content, relieves constipation, making it a natural laxative. Take one tablespoonful of molasses in a glass of milk. Always make sure that you rinse your mouth or better still, brush your teeth afterwards to prevent tooth decay.

Bran

The fibrous coating of the wheatgrain, bran is an inexpensive way of including roughage in the diet. It is rich in aneurin (vitamin B_1), a deficiency of which can cause poor elimination. It also contains protein, calcium, iron and vitamins in appreciable amounts.

The coarse bran composed of large particles is the most effective in treating constipation. Start by taking two teaspoonfuls twice a day and gradually increase the dose to two tablespoonfuls twice or three times a day. Flatulence can occur but it soon passes once bran has become a part of the daily diet.

Wheatgerm

High in the B vitamins and other nutrients, this cereal is an excellent starter for lazy bowels and nutritionally depleted bodies.

Sprinkle one tablespoon of wheatgerm on cereals and salads and into fruit juices, soups, and stews just before serving.

Yogurt (plain)

The healthy bacteria in yogurt utilizes the sugar in milk and converts it into lactic acid which helps to produce soft stools that are eliminated easily without straining.

Pour over breakfast cereals, fruit salad, or simply enjoy it by itself.

A HIGH-FIBRE START TO THE DAY

Orange, grapefruit or pineapple (whole or fresh juice)
followed by
dried apricots with chopped apple, wheatgerm and milk or yogurt
or prunes with chopped banana, bran and milk or yogurt
or porridge with raisins, wheatgerm and milk

or muesli with chopped figs, sunflower seeds, bran and milk or yogurt
or yogurt with chopped pear, wheatgerm and molasses
followed by
wholegrain toast and honey
or bran crispbread and honey
followed by
milk or fruit juice with brewer's yeast

THE INTERNAL CLEANSING PLAN

Are you working too hard, worrying too much, eating too many 'convenience' foods and exercising, relaxing and sleeping too little? Are you feeling tense, tired, 'tubby', sluggish and unable to cope? If the answer is in the affirmative, you could benefit tremendously from the Internal Cleansing Plan. This spring-clean, which is beneficial both physically and psychologically, doesn't involve fasting or anything even remotely unpleasant, but is a programme that pampers and detoxifies your system, making you look and feel like a new person. A fortune spent on creams and potions might make you feel good to begin with, but it is only a temporary fillip that is unlikely to result in any long-term benefit. However, with the Internal Cleansing Plan, the emphasis is on drinking lots of liquid to flush out impurities and eating fresh, wholesome, delicious foods high in fibre and natural vitamins which, when raw, possess remarkable properties that improve cellular activity, increase energy, and protect the body from premature ageing and the illnesses associated with advancing years.

For this cleansing programme you need between thirty-six hours and several days when you can be alone. If your partner is going away on business, arrange for the children to stay with grandparents at the same time. Single people living alone can arrange days to suit themselves and weekends usually are the most convenient time.

For the days ahead you will need to stock up with fresh fruits and plenty of them, particularly grapes, lemons, oranges, pineapple, grapefruits, and water melon, vegetable and salad ingredients such as avocados, lettuce, cabbage, parsley, watercress, tomatoes, peppers (green, red and yellow), cucumber, onions, celery, carrots etc., not forgetting sunflower, pumpkin and sesame seeds. Check that you have enough vitamins and wonder foods like cod-liver oil or capsules, brewer's yeast containing all the B vitamins, calcium tablets, low-fat dried and semi-skimmed or skimmed milk, wheatgerm, yogurt (plain) and blackstrap molasses.

Water is a marvellous internal cleanser that helps to slow down the ageing process and therefore is an important part of the treatment. Our body cells are composed almost entirely of water, but tea, coffee and alcohol consumed in large quantities actually dehydrate the cells, thus causing them to die prematurely. Replenishing the body's natural fluids helps to maintain young, healthy cells. Drink a large glassful of tepid mineral water first thing in the morning and throughout the day now and every day of your life.

Day 1

On awakening
1   Lie back and stretch your muscles several times like a cat, and then flex your joints. Now you are toned up and ready to start the day
2   Drink a large glass of tepid mineral water, with lemon if desired

Breakfast
1 orange and 1 lemon juiced and topped up with tepid mineral water
followed by
a slice of water melon, sprinkled with ginger if desired
or a slice of pineapple
followed by
yogurt mixed with a chopped apple (unpeeled), sunflower seeds, bran (2 tablespoonfuls), wheatgerm (1 tablespoonful) and blackstrap molasses (1 teaspoonful)
followed by
a glass of mineral water, with lemon if desired
or a cup of herbal tea with lemon
immediately after eating take
fish-liver oil or capsules, the equivalent of 5,000iu (vitamin A) and 400iu (vitamin D)
brewer's yeast, the equivalent of 2 teaspoonfuls
calcium (800mg)

After breakfast
Plan your beauty treatments for the day. Remember to include hair conditioning, skin cleansing using a face mask and a scrub, toning and moisturizing, face and body depilatory, and nails, hands and feet treatments

Midday
Nibble on several pieces of fruit of your choice (not bananas)
followed by
a glass of tepid mineral water, with lemon if desired

Lunch
Chicken, fish or liver (grilled)
with salad consisting of diced carrot, onion, celery, cabbage, avocado, parsley and

sunflower seeds with either vegetable oil (cold pressed) and lemon juice or cider vinegar or yogurt and avocado blended together
followed by
a glass of tepid mineral water, with lemon if desired
or a cup of herbal tea with lemon

Mid afternoon
Go for a brisk walk in a park or any green, open space
on returning
nibble on several pieces of fruit of your choice (not bananas)
followed by
a glass of tepid mineral water, with lemon if desired

Early Evening (about 6pm, not later)
Chicken, fish or liver (grilled)
with salad consisting of lettuce, tomato, pepper, cucumber, spring onions, watercress and sunflower, sesame and pumpkin seeds and nuts (unsalted) with either vegetable oil (cold pressed) and lemon juice or cider vinegar, or yogurt and avocado blended together

Before retiring
1   Take a bath. Add a cupful of cider vinegar and two tablespoons of vegetable oil to the warm (not hot) water. The cider vinegar which removes impurities and dead skin cells, has a wonderfully relaxing effect. The oil coats the body in a fine, lubricating film, thus preventing sebum in excessive amounts from being washed away. It is a good body moisturizer too
2   Gently loofah your body
3   Whilst soaking, sip the molasses drink (1 teaspoonful of blackstrap molasses dissolved in a cup of fortified milk)
4   Rinse all over with cooler water before towelling dry
5   Brush your teeth thoroughly. Molasses is a rich source of nutrients, but like all sugar, if allowed to coat the teeth, it can cause dental problems

Day 2
As Day 1

3
Weight

Ideal Weight Chart for Women of Thirty and Over

Height		Small Frame		Medium Frame		Large Frame	
ft. in.	*cm*	*lb*	*kg*	*lb*	*kg*	*lb*	*kg*
4' 8"	142	86– 92	39–42	90–101	41–46	98–113	44–51
4' 9"	145	89– 96	40–43	93–105	42–47	100–116	45–52
4' 10"	147	92– 98	42–44	96–108	44–49	103–119	46–54
4' 11"	150	94–101	43–46	99–111	45–50	107–122	48–55
5' 0"	152	96–104	44–47	102–114	46–52	110–125	50–57
5' 1"	155	98–107	45–48	105–117	47–53	112–129	51–58
5' 2"	157	101–110	46–50	108–120	49–54	115–132	52–60
5' 3"	160	104–113	47–51	111–124	50–56	119–136	54–61
5' 4"	163	107–116	48–52	113–127	51–57	123–139	56–63
5' 5"	165	110–119	50–54	116–130	52–59	126–142	57–64
5' 6"	168	113–123	51–56	119–135	54–61	129–146	58–66
5' 7"	170	117–127	53–57	124–140	56–63	133–150	60–68
5' 8"	173	121–131	55–59	129–144	58–65	137–155	62–70
5' 9"	175	125–135	57–61	133–149	60–67	142–160	64–72
5' 10"	178	129–140	58–63	136–152	61–69	146–164	66–74
5' 11"	180	133–145	60–66	140–155	63–70	150–169	68–76
6' 0"	183	137–149	62–67	144–159	65–72	153–173	69–78

YOUR IDEAL WEIGHT

You know how much you weigh, but how heavy should you be? Study the chart below according to your height and body frame (no cheating now) and see what your weight ought to be. As for myself, I am 5′7¼″ tall, big-boned, over thirty by decades rather than years, and weigh 147lb. As you can see, I am no feather-weight, but I am within the weight range that is considered ideal. How about you?

Ideal Weight Chart for Men of Thirty and Over

Height		Small Frame		Medium Frame		Large Frame	
ft. in.	cm	lb	kg	lb	kg	lb	kg
5′ 2″	157	112–120	51–54	118–129	53–58	126–141	57–64
5′ 3″	160	115–123	52–56	121–132	55–60	129–144	58–65
5′ 4″	163	118–126	53–57	124–135	56–61	132–148	60–67
5′ 5″	165	121–129	55–58	127–139	57–63	135–152	61–69
5′ 6″	168	124–133	56–60	130–143	59–65	138–156	62–71
5′ 7″	170	128–137	58–62	134–147	61–66	142–161	64–73
5′ 8″	173	132–141	60–64	138–151	62–68	146–166	66–75
5′ 9″	175	136–145	61–66	142–156	64–71	151–170	68–77
5′ 10″	178	140–150	63–68	146–160	66–72	155–175	70–79
5′ 11″	180	144–154	65–70	150–165	68–75	159–179	72–81
6′ 0″	183	148–158	67–71	154–170	70–77	163–184	74–83
6′ 1″	185	152–162	69–73	158–175	71–79	168–189	76–85
6′ 2″	187	156–166	71–75	162–180	73–81	173–194	78–88
6′ 3″	190	160–171	72–77	167–185	75–84	177–199	80–90
6′ 4″	193	164–176	74–80	172–190	78–86	182–204	82–92

CALORIES

A calorie is simply a unit of measure needed to produce energy. Calories are being burned up constantly but the exact number needed to meet the bodily requirements of the individual varies from person to person. Here is a formula to assess approximately one's calorie requirements.

First write down your ideal body weight, that is to say the weight at which you feel, look and perform your best (see Ideal Weight Charts). For example, supposing you are 5'6" (1.68m) tall, of medium frame, with an ideal body weight of 122lb (55kg; 1lb is equal to 0.45kg). Begin by multiplying that number by 15. If you are between the ages of 18 and 35, add 200 to the figure arrived at. If you are between 35 and 55, neither add nor subtract anything. Those who are between 55 and 75 should subtract 300. This final figure is approximately the number of calories needed to maintain ideal weight for the individual who leads a fairly active life.

$$
\begin{array}{rl}
\text{Ideal Weight} & 122 \text{ lb} \\
\times & 15 \\
\hline
& 1{,}830 \text{ calories}
\end{array}
$$

$$
\begin{array}{lcl}
\text{Aged } 18\text{–}35 \ (+200) & = & 2{,}030 \text{ calories} \\
\text{Aged } 35\text{–}55 \ (\text{nil}) & = & 1{,}830 \text{ calories} \\
\text{Aged } 55\text{–}75 \ (-300) & = & 1{,}530 \text{ calories}
\end{array}
$$

WEIGHT LOSS

A person's normal capacity to eat is related partly to build, a tall man having a slightly larger stomach capacity than a short woman. But an habitual over-eater increases the stomach's capacity for food to such an extent that it continues to crave for the quantity and the type of foods it is accustomed to, until it is disciplined and satisfied with a normal daily intake of good-quality food. Food intake that exceeds the body's requirements is processed, converted, and duly stored as body fat.

The Psychology of Weight Loss

Do
- Chew your food slowly. Not only will you enjoy the food more, but you will feel satisfied with smaller portions

- Eat only when you feel hungry and never for the sake of it
- Begin by eating the meat, fish, fowl or liver and green vegetables. By the time you have finished, the chances are that you won't want the potatoes after all
- Try to arrange it so that you sit down to the main meal preferably mid-day or as early in the evening as possible. The calories from foods eaten early in the day are more likely to be burned-up and not converted into fat
- Nibble on fruits and raw vegetables whenever you feel peckish. The high fibre content will eliminate hunger pangs. Plain yogurt also has the same effect
- Take a teaspoonful of either honey or diabetic jam or marmalade when the urge for something sweet is irresistible
- Always 'think thin'. By doing so you will minimize the craving for sugary, fattening foods

Don't
- Blame your glands for your weight problem
- Skip breakfast in the hope that it will help you shed unwanted pounds. What it will do is make you feel hungry later in the morning and the calorie consumption is likely to be far greater than if you had started the day with a lightly boiled egg and a slice of wholegrain bread
- Dress up salads or vegetables with creamy sauces, butter, salad cream or mayonnaise. Keep to a simple oil (preferably cold pressed) and lemon juice or cider vinegar dressing
- Serve your meal on a large dinner plate, but one several sizes smaller. It will make the portion look more like the one you were used to
- Eat the animal fats, sugar or salt found in processed and prepared foods, tinned meats and squashes
- Eat meals or snacks high in carbohydrate late at night. Unless you are a shift worker, the calories will be converted into fat
- Drink alcohol unless essential. Keep to pure fruit juices, or mineral water with a slice of lemon which at a social gathering is usually mistaken for gin and tonic

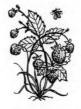

SEVEN-DAY WEIGHT-REDUCING AGELESS BEAUTY DIET

Day 1

Breakfast
Grapefruit or orange juice (freshly squeezed)
followed by
4 tablespoonfuls of muesli and nuts with ½ small banana and milk (low fat)
followed by
1 cup of milk (low fat)
or 1 cup of coffee (decaffeinated) with milk (low fat)
immediately after eating take
fish-liver oil or capsules, the equivalent of 5,000iu (vitamin A) and 400iu (vitamin D)
brewer's yeast, the equivalent of 2 teaspoonfuls
vitamin C (1,000mg)
wheatgerm oil or vitamin E capsules, the equivalent of 140iu
calcium (800mg)

Mid-morning
1 glass of celery or any liquidized vegetable juice
or 1 cup of milk (low fat)
or 12 tablespoons of yogurt (plain, fat-free and preferably homemade) flavoured with cinnamon or nutmeg
or 1 cup of tomato juice (liquidized in a blender)

Lunch
1 egg omelette (cooked in a little oil)
with a green salad tossed in lemon juice, and wheatgerm oil (2 teaspoonfuls)
followed by
yogurt (plain) with sunflower seeds (1 teaspoonful)
followed by
1 cup of tea with lemon

Tea 1 glass of vegetable juice

Dinner 4 oz (100g) of lean meat
with 1 leafy green vegetable (lightly steamed)
and tomato and sunflower seed salad (2 tomatoes and 1 tablespoonful sunflower seeds
tossed in 2 teaspoonfuls of vegetable oil, cold pressed)
followed by
1 cup of milk (low fat)
or 1 cup of tea with lemon or milk

Bedtime
1 cup of milk (hot or cold)

Day 2

Breakfast
Grapefruit or orange juice (freshly squeezed)
followed by
1 scrambled egg
with 2 wholemeal crackers
followed by
1 cup of milk (low fat)
or 1 cup of coffee (decaffeinated) with milk (low fat)
immediately after eating take
fish-liver oil or capsules, the equivalent of 5,000iu (vitamin A) and 400iu (vitamin D)
brewer's yeast, the equivalent of 2 teaspoonfuls
vitamin C (1,000mg)
wheatgerm oil or vitamin E capsules, the equivalent of 140iu
calcium (800mg)

Mid-morning
1 glass of celery or any vegetable juice (liquidized)
or 1 cup of milk (low fat)
or 12 tablespoons of yogurt (plain and fat-free) flavoured with cinnamon or nutmeg

Lunch
1 cup of tomato juice (liquidized in a blender)
followed by
fish (lightly grilled)
with wheatgerm (2 teaspoonfuls)
and a celery, tomato, carrot and cucumber salad tossed in 2 teaspoonfuls vegetable oil
(cold pressed) and lemon juice

followed by
12 tablespoons of yogurt (flavoured with cinnamon or nutmeg)
followed by
a cup of tea with lemon

Tea
a glass of vegetable juice (liquidized in a blender)

Dinner
Liver (grilled lightly)
with cabbage, red and green pepper salad tossed in lemon juice or a little oil (cold pressed)
followed by
1 cup of milk (low fat)
or 1 cup of tea with lemon or milk (low fat)

Bedtime
1 cup of milk (hot or cold)

Day 3

Breakfast
Grapefruit or orange juice (freshly squeezed)
followed by
1 poached egg
with 2 wholemeal crackers
followed by
1 cup of milk (low fat)
or 1 cup of coffee (decaffeinated) with milk (low fat)
immediately after eating take
fish-liver oil or capsules, the equivalent of 5,000iu (vitamin A) and 400iu (vitamin D)
brewer's yeast, the equivalent of 2 teaspoonfuls
vitamin C (1,000mg)
wheatgerm oil or vitamin E capsules, the equivalent of 140iu
calcium (800mg)

Mid-morning
1 glass of celery or any vegetable juice (liquidized)
or 1 cup of milk (low fat)
or 12 tablespoons of yogurt (plain, fat-free) flavoured with cinnamon or nutmeg

Lunch
1 apple
followed by
a mixed salad (no potatoes)
with cottage cheese
and wheatgerm (2 teaspoonfuls)
followed by
a piece of fruit (not bananas)
or 12 tablespoons of yogurt (fat-free)
with sunflower seeds,
or fresh raspberries or strawberries
followed by
1 cup of tea with lemon
or 1 cup of coffee (decaffeinated) with milk

Tea
1 glass of tomato or any vegetable juice

Dinner
Chicken (grilled and skinned)
with a green, leafy vegetable (lightly steamed)
and a salad of your choice
followed by
1 cup of milk (low fat)
or 1 cup of tea with lemon or milk (low fat)

Bedtime
1 cup of milk (hot or cold)

Day 4

Breakfast
Grapefruit or orange juice (freshly squeezed)
followed by
2 tablespoonfuls of porridge or oatmeal cooked with water
with 2 teaspoonfuls sunflower seeds
and 1 teaspoonful blackstrap molasses
and milk (low fat)
followed by
1 cup milk (low fat)

or 1 cup of coffee (decaffeinated) with milk (low fat)
immediately after eating take
fish-liver oil or capsules, the equivalent of 5,000iu (vitamin A) and 400iu (vitamin D)
brewer's yeast, the equivalent of 2 teaspoonfuls
vitamin C (1,000mg)
wheatgerm oil or vitamin E capsules, the equivalent of 140iu
calcium (800mg)

Mid-morning
1 glass of celery or any vegetable juice
or 1 cup of milk (low fat)
or 12 tablespoons of yogurt (plain and fat-free) flavoured with cinnamon or nutmeg

Lunch
1 glass of tomato juice (fresh)
or 1 apple
followed by
shrimps
with mixed salad
followed by
yogurt (plain and fat-free)
with sunflower seeds
and wheatgerm (2 teaspoonfuls)
or a piece of fruit (not bananas)
followed by
1 cup of tea with lemon

Tea
1 glass of tomato or any vegetable juice

Dinner
Soup (clear), preferably homemade
followed by
fish (grilled)
with green salad
followed by
1 cup of milk (low fat)
or 1 cup of tea with lemon or milk (low fat)

Bedtime
1 cup of milk (hot or cold)

Day 5

Breakfast
Grapefruit or orange juice (freshly squeezed)
followed by
1 slice of granary or wholewheat toast
with cheese
followed by
1 cup of milk (low fat)
or 1 cup of coffee (decaffeinated) with milk (low fat)
immediately after eating take
fish-liver oil or capsules, the equivalent of 5,000iu (vitamin A) and 400iu (vitamin D)
brewer's yeast, the equivalent of 2 teaspoonfuls
vitamin C (1,000mg)
wheatgerm oil or vitamin E capsules, the equivalent of 140iu
calcium (800mg)

Mid-morning
1 glass of celery or any vegetable juice
or 12 tablespoons of yogurt (plain and fat-free) flavoured with cinnamon or nutmeg
or 1 cup of milk (low fat)

Lunch
1 glass of tomato juice (fresh)
or a piece of fruit (not bananas)
followed by
liver (grilled)
with either 2 vegetables consisting of one green, leafy one (lightly steamed)
or a salad of your choice
and wheatgerm (2 teaspoonfuls)
followed by
yogurt (plain and fat-free) flavoured with cinnamon or nutmeg
followed by
1 cup of tea with lemon

Tea
1 glass of tomato or any vegetable juice (fresh)

Dinner
Chicken or game (grilled)
with 1 green, leafy vegetable (lightly steamed)
and mixed salad
followed by
1 cup of milk (low fat)
or 1 cup of tea with lemon or milk (low fat)

Bedtime
1 cup of milk (low fat), hot or cold

Day 6

Breakfast
Grapefruit or orange juice (fresh)
followed by
1 slice of granary or wholemeal toast
with honey
or muesli
with milk (low fat)
followed by
1 cup of milk (low fat)
or 1 cup of coffee (decaffeinated) with milk (low fat)
immediately after eating take
fish-liver oil or capsules, the equivalent of 5,000iu (vitamin A) and 400iu (vitamin D)
brewer's yeast, the equivalent of 2 teaspoonfuls
vitamin C (1,000mg)
wheatgerm oil or vitamin E capsules, the equivalent of 140iu
calcium (800mg)

Mid-morning
1 glass of celery or any vegetable juice
or 1 cup of milk (low fat)
or 12 tablespoons of yogurt (plain and fat-free)
with wheatgerm and sunflower seeds

Lunch
1 cup of tomato juice
or 1 apple

followed by
cream cheese (low fat)
with salad of your choice
followed by
12 tablespoons of yogurt (plain and fat-free)
with 1 tablespoon fresh fruit
followed by
1 cup of tea with lemon

Tea
1 glass of tomato or any vegetable juice

Dinner
Brown rice (2 tablespoonfuls)
with soya beans
and sunflower seeds (2 teaspoonfuls)
and tomato salad
followed by
1 cup of milk (low fat)
or 1 cup of tea with lemon or milk (low fat)

Bedtime
1 cup of milk (low fat) hot or cold

Day 7

Breakfast
Grapefruit or orange juice (fresh)
followed by
sardines on wholewheat crackers
or cream cheese (fat free) on wholewheat crackers
followed by
1 cup of milk (low fat)
or 1 cup of coffee (decaffeinated) with milk (low fat)
immediately after eating take
fish-liver oil or capsules, the equivalent of 5,000iu (vitamin A) and 400iu (vitamin D)
brewer's yeast, the equivalent of 2 teaspoonfuls
vitamin C (1,000mg)
wheatgerm oil or vitamin E capsules, the equivalent of 140iu
calcium (800mg)

Mid-morning
1 glass of celery or any vegetable juice
or 1 cup of milk (low fat)
or 12 tablespoons of yogurt (plain and fat free) flavoured with cinnamon or nutmeg

Lunch
1 cup of tomato juice
or a piece of fruit (not bananas)
followed by
4oz (100g) of lean meat
with 2 cooked vegetables consisting of 1 green, leafy one (lightly steamed)
or tomato and green pepper salad
followed by
yogurt (plain and fat free) with wheatgerm (2 teaspoonfuls)
followed by
1 cup of tea with lemon or milk (low fat)

Tea
1 glass of tomato or any vegetable juice

Dinner
Soup (clear), preferably homemade
or 1 apple
followed by
meat loaf
with 2 vegetables consisting of 1 green, leafy one (lightly steamed)
or salad of your choice
followed by
1 cup of milk (low fat)
or 1 cup of tea with lemon or milk (low fat)

Bedtime
1 cup of milk (low fat), hot or cold

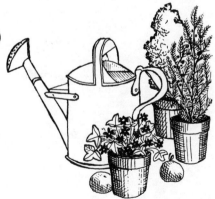

WEIGHT-REDUCING HEALTH JUICES

Fresh Vegetable Juice Cocktail

1 part carrot
1 part celery

Put the ingredients in a liquidizer, cover with water and blend until smooth. This slimming aid with its high sodium content is also recommended for arthritis and the nervous system.

Slimmer's Delight

3 parts carrot
1 part spinach

Put the ingredients in a liquidizer, cover with water and blend until smooth. An excellent internal cleanser that is particularly helpful to those who are overweight.

Salad Surprise

6 parts carrot
5 parts cucumber
3 parts beetroot

Put the ingredients in a liquidizer, cover with water and blend until smooth. A superb weight-reducing cleanser and healer.

Cool Cucumber

3 parts cucumber
1 part apple

Put the ingredients in a liquidizer, cover with water, and blend until smooth. The juices of cucumber, a natural diuretic, and apple combine to promote intestinal activity and tone and cleanse the system.

Vegetable Slim

8 parts carrot
5 parts celery
3 parts cucumber

Put the ingredients in a liquidizer, cover with water and blend until smooth.

Fat Foe

6 parts carrot
5 parts apple
5 parts cabbage

Put the ingredients in a liquidizer, cover with water and blend until smooth.

Anita Special

Put the ingredients in a liquidizer, cover with water and blend until smooth. High in sulphur and choline that cleanses the intestinal tract and helps those fighting the 'flab'. Its rich vitamin C content fights infection. Drinking cabbage juice either by itself or combined with other juices may produce gas, but this is an indication that the intestinal 'flora' is not as healthy as it should be, so persevere and the intestines will become more efficient at assimilating this juice.

6 parts carrot
5 parts cabbage
3 parts spinach

Celery Cocktail

Put the ingredients in a liquidizer, cover with water and blend until smooth.

15 parts celery
1 part grapefruit

Note Each part is a measure by volume not weight. These weight-reducing health juices are an effective way of losing weight, but only when used as part of a carefully controlled diet. For more information on Fruit and Vegetable Juices, turn to page 25.

UNDER WEIGHT?

If you are slim be grateful and make sure that you stay that way. However, if you are painfully thin and feel unwell, it is advisable to do something about it; looking gaunt and haggard is just as unattractive as being excessively overweight.

Gaining weight does not necessitate gorging on high-carbohydrate, low-protein foods as one would imagine, but including delicious, body-building foods, high in protein and calcium, and the B vitamins to enable those who are tense and highly strung to relax.

The following menu will improve your appearance, but more important still, should improve your health and make you feel better too.

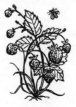

WEIGHT-GAINING MENU GUIDE

Breakfast
A glass of orange, pineapple or grapefruit juice (fresh)
followed by
1 egg (poached or scrambled)
with 1 slice of granary or wholegrain bread
or porridge with honey or blackstrap molasses and milk
or muesli with wheatgerm, honey and milk
followed by
2 slices of granary or wholegrain toast with margarine and honey or blackstrap molasses
or cheese or peanut butter
followed by
a glass of milk with wheatgerm
followed by
coffee with milk
or tea with milk ⎫ If desired

Mid-morning
a glass of milk (fortified)
or a glass of carrot juice (fresh)
or yogurt (plain) with brewer's yeast and honey or blackstrap molasses

Lunch
A cup of vegetable soup
followed by
carrot, avocado, raisin and sunflower seed salad with peanut oil dressing (see recipe p. 83)
or prawn or shrimp salad with celery, and avocado and peanut oil dressing
or banana, orange, raisin and sunflower seed salad with peanut oil dressing
or two scrambled eggs on granary or wholegrain bread (if eggs were not eaten at breakfast)
or cottage or cream cheese with granary or wholegrain bread
followed by
fruit salad (fresh) with nuts and yogurt
or yogurt (plain) with banana and honey or blackstrap molasses
followed by
a glass of milk (fortified)
or tea with milk or lemon

Tea
A glass of milk (fortified)
or banana milk (see page 84)
or nutty, sunflower milk (see page 84)

Dinner
A cup of fruit or vegetable juice (fresh)
followed by
meat (lean)
or liver
or fish   } preferably grilled
or fowl
with potatoes (jacketed or boiled) with yogurt (plain) or margarine
and green salad with peanut oil dressing
or any two vegetables of your choice, consisting of one green, leafy one (lightly steamed)
followed by
fresh or stewed fruit
or baked apple with raisins
and honey and yogurt (if desired)
followed by
tea with lemon (small cup)
or coffee with milk (small cup)

Bedtime
A glass of milk (fortified)
or banana milk
or yogurt (plain) with wheatgerm
with calcium, brewer's yeast and other vitamin and mineral supplements

Recipes

Peanut Oil Salad Dressing

Blend all the ingredients together until smooth. Pour into a bottle with a screw-type lid and refrigerate.

1 pint (570ml) peanut oil
½ pint (285ml) lemon juice or cider vinegar
1 teaspoonful mustard (french)
honey (to taste)
seasalt (to taste)

Banana Milk

1 banana (large and very ripe)
1 pint (570ml) milk
honey or blackstrap molasses (to taste)

Place all the ingredients in a liquidizer and blend until smooth.

Nutty, Sunflower Milk

2oz (50 gram) mixed nuts (unsalted)
1 pint (570ml) milk
honey (to taste)

Place the nuts in a coffee mill and grind to a fine consistency. Then, place the nuts, milk and honey in a liquidizer and blend until smooth.

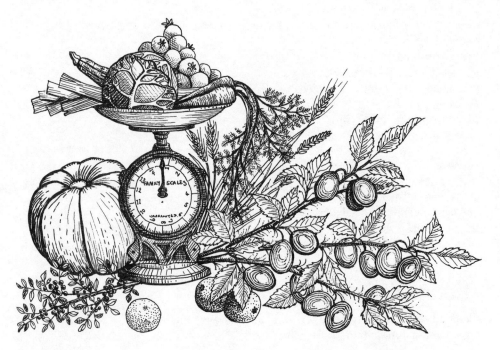

4
Sleep

Rest, in a state of complete relaxation, is necessary if we are to function efficiently and look our best. Unfortunately, rest that culminates in sleep can become increasingly difficult as problems, doubts and fears increase, and even when we do sleep, the more anxious and tense we are, the less chance we have of reaching the depth of unconsciousness necessary to feel refreshed.

Once in bed, don't be a slave to anxiety. Put it to sleep until the morning. Now position yourself comfortably. The foetus position, lying curled up on your side is believed to be the most restful, but I find that lying flat on my back, without pillows, can also be very relaxing.

Now concentrate on unwinding your muscles. First, flex and relax your feet, then ankles, calves, thighs, arms, hands, neck and back. You'll be surprised at the number of muscles that are tense. The next stage, which requires more controlled, conscious thought, is to empty your mind of ideas, thoughts, and images, however vague, transient and insignificant. Try to visualize your mind as a large, black screen that must be kept blank. Push away any 'picture' immediately it appears. As the gaps between the pictures lengthen, so sleep will eclipse further thoughts.

NATURAL AIDS TO SLEEP

1   Go for brisk walks in green, open areas during the day and in the evening, if possible, for fresh air is a natural tranquillizer

2 Take a slow, relaxing, warm bath before retiring (see page 160)
3 Drink a glass of warm milk before bed. It may sound old-fashioned, but it works. Avoid tea, coffee, alcohol and other strong stimulants
4 For insomniacs, take two or three calcium or vitamin B$_6$ tablets in the form of brewer's yeast or the B complex group with a milky or other sleep-inducing nightcap (see page 88)
5 Read a good book in bed before turning off the light
6 Sleep with a bedroom window partially open

MENU TO AID SLEEP

Breakfast
Fruit or fruit juice (fresh)
followed by
egg with wholegrain bread
or wholegrain cereal with wheatgerm and milk, yogurt (plain) or buttermilk
followed by
milk (preferably fortified)
or buttermilk
or coffee (decaffeinated) made with milk

Mid-morning
Yogurt (plain)
or milk
or buttermilk
with calcium tablets, the equivalent of 300mg

Lunch
Salad with cottage or cheddar cheese
followed by
egg custard
or milk pudding
or buttermilk
or yogurt (plain)
and/or milk

Mid-afternoon
Milk
or tomato juice
with calcium tablets, the equivalent of 300mg
and brewer's yeast, the equivalent of 2 teaspoonfuls

Dinner
Fruit or vegetable juice
followed by
liver (grilled)
or fish (grilled or poached)
or meat (lean)
or fowl
with two cooked vegetables consisting of one green, leafy one (lightly steamed)
followed by
yogurt (plain) with fresh fruit
or cheese with wholewheat crackers
or milk

Before Retiring
A hot, milky drink, preferably made with fortified milk
or another sleep-inducing nightcap
with calcium tablets, the equivalent of 400mg
and brewer's yeast, the equivalent of 2 teaspoonfuls

Note   This menu, which is designed specifically to ensure a good night's sleep when all else fails, can be tried for several days at a time. Thereafter, it is best to move on to the Stress-Reducing Menu.

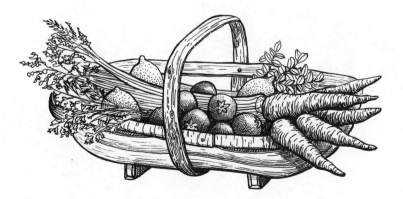

87

SLEEP-INDUCING NIGHTCAPS

Sleeptime Special

½ pint (285ml) hot
milk (preferably
fortified)
1 tablespoon dried
milk (skimmed)
2 teaspoonfuls
blackstrap
molasses
2 teaspoonfuls
brewer's yeast

Dissolve the molasses in a little warm water, add the dried milk and stir well. Add the hot milk and the brewer's yeast and stir thoroughly.

This Sleeptime Special induces peaceful sleep, from which you should awaken quite refreshed.

Molasses Milk

½ pint (285ml) hot
milk (preferably
fortified)
2 teaspoonfuls
blackstrap
molasses

Add the molasses to the hot milk and stir until it is dissolved.

This milk is an excellent aid to restful sleep.

Bergamot Milk

½ tablespoonful
bergamot leaves
(dried)
¼ pint (140ml) hot
milk (preferably
fortified)
honey (to taste)

Pour the hot milk over the leaves and leave to infuse for seven minutes. Then, strain and add the honey.

Red Clover Tea

1oz (25 grams) red
clover flowers
(fresh)
1 pint (570ml)
boiling water

Pour the boiling water over the flowers and leave to infuse for twenty minutes. Strain.

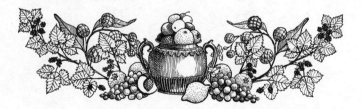

Chamomile Tea

Pour the boiling water over the flowers and leave to infuse for fifteen to twenty minutes. Strain.

½oz (12 grams)
chamomile flowers
(fresh) or
¼oz (6 grams)
chamomile flowers
(dried)
1 pint boiling water

Grapefruit Cocktail

Dissolve the molasses in a little hot water. Stir the molasses liquid and the brewer's yeast into the grapefruit juice.

1 glass warm
grapefruit juice
(fresh)
2 teaspoonfuls
blackstrap
molasses
1 teaspoonful
brewer's yeast

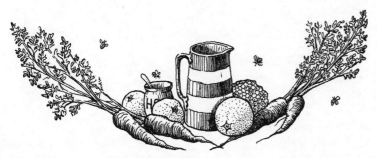

5

Stress

Controlled stress is an integral part of modern life. Uncontrolled, it can be a killer. Stress inhibits digestion and causes gastric ulcers, migraine, insomnia, and high blood pressure to name but a few illnesses. It also quickly depletes the vitamin C stored in the adrenal glands, which results in a destruction of tissues and a greater susceptibility to infections and diseases. Consequently, massive intakes of vitamin C are advisable.

Obviously, a diet specifically designed to enable the body to cope with a period of stress is vital (see page 92), but unless you learn to conserve and not waste nervous energy, you will never learn the secret of agelessness.

All of us experience stress of one kind or another every day, but it is important to channel that nervous energy in a productive way, so significantly reducing the potentially harmful effects of stress.

Once drugs were thought to be the only way to cope with stress. Now, scientists have found that the ability to release excessive stress is within all of us, provided we know how. Here are some simple and easy ways of reducing stress to levels of safety that are unlikely to endanger health.

WAYS OF COPING WITH STRESS

- Talk out problems in a constructive and logical way with a companion, relative or close friend who can be trusted
- Give vent to anger in physical activity such as gardening, exercising, walking, jogging,

swimming or some favourite sport. If you need to work off anger in a verbal way, go to a place where there is no chance of being overheard and speak or shriek your mind! It will enable you to give vent to your frustrations without having to cope with recriminations and repercussions afterwards

- Take a warm and relaxing bath (see page 160)
- Find time to pause. Go to a park, a river, or a green, open and tranquil place to pause and listen to the birds, water etc., and enjoy the wonders of nature
- Take up a hobby that is pleasurable. My hobby is fish-keeping, which is wonderfully relaxing
- If you can't change the situation, learn to accept it. Remember that tragedy and bad luck are cross-roads over which we must all travel to a better and a happier life
- Take one worry and one day at a time. Forget about the troubles that may be ahead. They may never happen!
- Don't waste energy on trivia. Concentrate on important issues and discard the rest

Another quick way to relieve tension during the day, and a favourite of mine, which only takes a few minutes is to sit up straight on an upright chair near an open window. Close your eyes and breathe deeply and slowly. Now think of a pastime that you find particularly relaxing – walking in woods, listening to birds, watching a running stream, fishing, sunbathing on golden sands – anything that makes you feel really peaceful and lets your mind float. My mental image is sitting near a stream or river. Still with your eyes closed, breathing deeply and concentrating on your own private daydream, choose a word which epitomizes this daydream, and quietly and slowly repeat the word, which in my case is 'water', 'water', 'water' . . . . Breathing slowly and deeply and releasing both mind and body in a daydream is wonderfully revitalizing.

THE SLANT-BOARD RELAXER

Standing on your head for several minutes each day is a superb muscle-relaxer. However, try as we might, most of us, myself included, are unable to elevate ourselves into an upside-down position, and by trying it, one runs the risk of injury.

A safer, easier and effective technique is the Slant-Board Relaxer. This consists of an ordinary, solid piece of wood, eighteen inches wide and about six feet long, although it will need to be longer if you are extremely tall. Place a stool or a solid piece of furniture that is no more than fifteen inches high, against a wall and wedge one end of the slant-board on it so that it cannot slip. Now lie on the board with your feet raised and your head near the floor. This yoga position, with the board for support, straightens the spine, relaxes the muscles, relieves the pressure on puffy, swollen legs, ankles and feet, while the increased flow of blood to the face, scalp and brain stimulates the complexion, hair and enables the brain to function faster and more efficiently. Arlene Dahl, one of the real beauties of Hollywood said that 'twenty minutes on a slant-board is equivalent to two hours of sleep. If you do this daily, you'll never need a face-lift'.

Begin by using the slant-board for a minute or two daily, gradually increasing the time spent by one minute each day until you can recline quite comfortably for fifteen minutes twice a day or whenever you feel tired and unable to cope.

STRESS-REDUCING MENU

Breakfast
An orange or fresh fruit juice
followed by
either ¼lb (100 grams) liver (grilled lightly) as part of a mixed grill
or fish as part of a mixed grill
or cheese omelette
or eggs (scrambled with powdered, skimmed milk)
or cheese on granary or wholegrain bread
or porridge cooked with milk and topped with wheatgerm and sunflower seeds
followed by
granary or wholegrain toast topped with
either cheese
or peanut butter
or blackstrap molasses
followed by
a fortified milk drink (see page 16), but no tea or coffee
immediately after eating take
fish-liver oil or capsules, the equivalent of 5,000iu (vitamin A) and 400iu (vitamin D)
B_2 (20mg) and B_6 (20mg) contained in brewer's yeast or the B complex group
vitamin C (1,000mg)
wheatgerm oil or vitamin E capsules between 140 and 200iu
calcium (600mg)

Mid-morning
Fruit or vegetable juice or fortified milk drink to which has been added 2 teaspoonfuls brewer's yeast
or 16 tablespoons of yogurt (plain) with 1 teaspoonful blackstrap molasses

Lunch
Eggs (if none were eaten at breakfast)
or liver (grilled)
or fish
or fowl
or meat (lean)
followed by
fresh fruit of your choice
or nuts (unsalted) and seeds
followed by
fortified milk, buttermilk or yogurt (plain)
immediately after eating take
1 multi-vitamin and mineral tablet
1 teaspoonful (or the equivalent of) brewer's yeast
vitamin C (500mg)

with lightly steamed vegetables or
green salad tossed in oil (cold pressed)

Mid-afternoon
As for mid-morning

Dinner
Soup (homemade)
or vegetable juice
followed by
liver (grilled)
or meat (lean)
or fish
or fowl
or soya bean dish
followed by
fresh fruit
or yogurt (plain) with fresh fruit
or nuts (unsalted)
followed by
fortified milk
or buttermilk

with salad tossed in oil (cold pressed) or
lightly steamed green vegetables

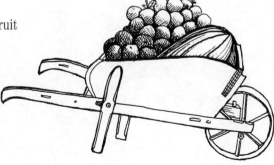

Bedtime
Fortified milk
or milky drink
or yogurt (plain) with blackstrap molasses
with brewer's yeast, the equivalent of 1 teaspoonful
1 multi-vitamin and mineral tablet
vitamin C (1,000mg)

If you are unable to take all the supplements in the quantities recommended or simply feel that you need a tonic, this vitamin-packed Liver Tonic costs next-to-nothing to make, and has none of the unpleasant taste associated with liver.

Liver Tonic

2 pints (1.15 litres)
vegetable juice or
clear, vegetable
soup
4 tablespoonfuls
liver (raw)
3 tablespoonfuls
parsley (fresh)
2 tablespoonfuls
spinach (fresh)
3 slices onion

Put all the ingredients in a liquidizer and blend until smooth. Take one glassful twice a day.

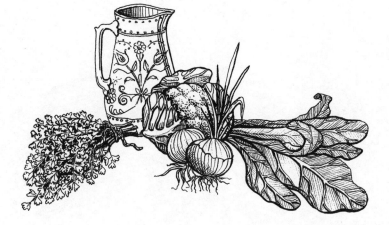

PART TWO

Natural Beauty from Top to Toe

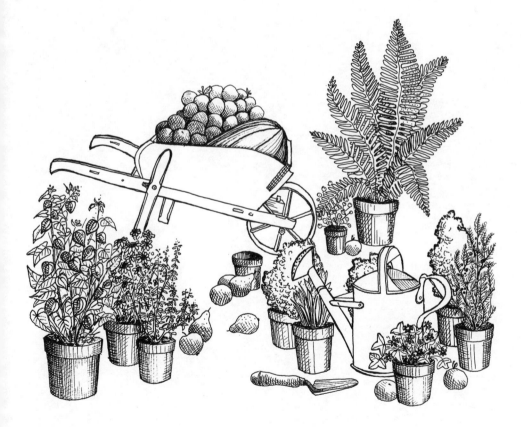

6
Skin

SKIN NUTRITION

Few people are blessed with perfect complexions. Most of us have to work at it, for skin needs good nutrition, vitamins and minerals, external nourishment, sleep, exercise, and fresh air to remain beautiful and blemish-free.

Skin is not an inanimate, cling-film-type covering but living tissue, consisting of billions of cells composed largely of protein and other nutrients. To function well and remain healthy, skin needs protein. When protein consumption exceeds skin and other body requirements, it is converted, temporarily, into stored protein from which supplies are replenished as the cells absorb the amino acids in the protein. As long as protein intake is adequate, the amino acid level remains constant, but if diet is neglected, stored reserves quickly become exhausted, thus resulting in wrinkles, loss of muscle tone, and the signs generally associated with ageing. For the best sources of protein turn to page 38.

Even with a sensible diet, vitamin and mineral supplements have an integral role to play, for they help to augment the nutrients in fresh foods, wholly or partially depleted by the effects of light, air, heat, cooking, handling, storing and freezing.

SYMPTOMS OF STARVATION

Deficiencies of individual vitamins manifest themselves in different ways. Dry, lined skin is common among women whose diets are lacking vitamin A. As cells die, they plug the pores, an accumulation of which appears as whiteheads and blackheads. Infection results in pimples. Vitamin A is formed from carotene found in carrots, apricots and all green vegetables. Other good sources of vitamin A and/or carotene are liver, fish liver oil, egg yolk and butter.

A common symptom of an acute vitamin B_2 deficiency is clearly visible as tiny wrinkles from the top lip upwards. Lipstick 'bleeds' producing an irregular, smudged appearance. However, if the deficiency is only slight but of long duration, the upper lip becomes progressively thinner until it is little more than a slit. The forehead, nose and chin take on an oily appearance and minute fatty deposits, similar to whiteheads, accumulate under the skin. Abnormally high colouration of the cheeks and across the nose, that on closer examination consists of a network of tiny blood vessels near the surface of the skin, is a condition known as 'acne rosacea'. Generally considered to be a sign of rude health, but in fact, more common among alcoholics, symptoms can disappear within a matter of weeks when nutrition is corrected and maximum absorption achieved. Intakes of liver, milk, yogurt, brewer's yeast, wheatgerm and other foods containing vitamin B_2 and other essential B vitamins should be increased. If a deficiency of one or more B vitamins occurs, a supplement containing all of them is required.

Wrinkles, loss of elasticity, brittle bones etc., are not a natural consequence of ageing, but indicative of inadequate vitamin C (ascorbic acid), which is essential in forming and maintaining collagen. To retain youthfulness, one's daily intake of ascorbic acid must be high enough to ensure saturation of the tissues, considered essential to health. When saturation occurs and the cells have all the vitamin C they need, any excess is excreted by the body. Fruits and fruit juices of lemons, oranges, and grapefruit, the richest and the most readily available sources of vitamin C, should be taken daily. Research into its regenerative powers showed that when patients who had undergone surgery were given four thousand milligrams of vitamin C daily, the healing process accelerated dramatically.

Another aid in healing damaged, burned and scarred skin tissue is vitamin E. Known as the 'anti-ageing vitamin', it is vital for the formation of body cells and connective tissue between them. Doctors in the USA have found that it helps in the treatment of many diseases, particularly in cases of blood clotting and where the oxygen supply is limited, as in coronary thrombosis, heart abnormalities, asthma etc. This vitamin occurs in several forms known as mixed tocopherols found in nuts, seeds, grains (whole), wheatgerm, bread (wholegrain) and cold-pressed oils.

The external application of essential oils absorbed through the outer layers of the skin helps to protect and preserve the connective tissues consisting of collagen (protein), so ensuring that healthy skin has form, firmness and resilience.

DRIED SKIN

Dried skin is a problem that increases with years, but underactive sebaceous glands, not age, are responsible.

The rate at which skin ages depends on genetic factors, general health and degrees of exposure to sun, wind, central heating, pollutants in the atmosphere and other environmental factors. A diet low in essential vitamins and minerals results in inadequate replacement of enzymes in the cells, which speeds up the degeneration associated with ageing.

In addition to ample nutrients, skin needs to be nourished with oils from fish and fish oil derivatives, cold-pressed vegetable oils, butter and nuts etc., to retain its smooth, plumped-up appearance. Evidence of too few such foods can be seen in the faces of women who keep to strict fat- and oil-free diets. By depriving their skin of essential oils, they are unbeknowingly sacrificing youthful complexions for prematurely wrinkled ones.

Cod-liver oil, rich in vitamins A and D and an excellent skin beautifier, is best taken in liquid, not capsule form. I agree that it has a disgusting smell, but take it as suggested on page 15 and you won't even notice it! Cod-liver oil applied externally also nourishes the skin and with the recipe on page 109 you can enjoy the benefits without the smell. Adding olive, sunflower, sesame, safflower, wheatgerm and other cold-pressed vegetable oils to salad dressings is a good way of helping to alleviate dried skin. Two tablespoonfuls of any cold-pressed oil taken daily, particularly if it is taken in addition to cod-liver oil, has a remarkable effect on skin and hair that is apparent within a matter of weeks.

Try to cut down on tea, coffee, and alcohol, which dehydrate skin cells, and replace them with mineral water and herbal teas. Mineral water detoxifies tissues, so helping to keep skin plumped-up, clear and beautiful.

The drying effect of central heating can be reduced by installing a humidifier. Alternatively, keep a container of water in every heated room or better still, an aquarium complete with fish and plants, which not only solves the problem of dry atmospheres but also helps alleviate stress.

OTHER AGEING FACTORS
Sun

Sun is the single most destructive force for drying and prematurely ageing the skin. The consequences of overexposure are apparent in any sun-bathing devotee; skin the thickness and texture of tanned leather that sags and is deeply wrinkled is the result of prolonged dehydration. Such old-looking skin does not appear overnight, but is the result of prolonged exposure over a period of years. To benefit from the sun without suffering the consequences, you need to understand how to sunbathe, if you must tan at all.

A high-protection sunscreen to screen out the harmful UV-B rays, overexposure to which results in burning, is vital, but a sunscreen product, however sophisticated, cannot protect the skin from cellular destruction and the degenerative changes in skin structure that result in premature ageing. The only safe way to maintain a youthful complexion is to stay out of the sun altogether. If, despite all warnings, you are still determined to tan, aim for a gentle one which is one or two shades deeper than your normal skin tone. Start by sunbathing for just ten minutes a day from between 9 and 11am and 3 and 5pm, when the sun's rays are less intense and therefore less likely to damage the skin, provided, of course, exposure is only for short periods at a time. Gradually increase exposure by five minutes each day.

Before sunbathing, take 1,000mg of PABA (contained in the B complex group of vitamins). Research shows that it increases one's tolerance to the sun without burning, but remember, it is unable to prevent damage on a cellular level.

Smoking

The dangers of smoking are well known. Lung cancer, emphysema, osteoporosis, heart and bronchial diseases are all directly related to this habit, but what smokers may not realize is that in addition to damaging health, smoking also ages the skin and rapidly too. The reason is that smoking robs the body of vitamin C, reserves of which would otherwise be available for the maintenance of healthy skin among other things. Dr W. J. McCormick of Canada discovered that one cigarette destroys 25mg of vitamin C, which means that a moderate smoker who averages twenty cigarettes a day is burning up vitamin C equivalent to that found in ten medium-sized oranges. An extensive study into the visible damage of smoking revealed that the skin of smokers ages up to twenty years earlier than non-smokers. So, a smoker of thirty-five is likely to have a complexion of a fifty-five year old non-smoker. 'Smoke Gets in your Eyes' is a sentimental and very charming song, but the realities are neither romantic nor particularly attractive. For the very act of smoking encourages wrinkles. Squinting causes lines around the eyes and puckering of the lips accentuates lip creases, particularly visible on the upper lip into which lipstick 'bleeds'. Carbon monoxide also harms the skin in another way by constricting the veins and reducing circulation, thus resulting in progressively drier skin.

Alcohol

Alcohol robs the body of the B vitamins (needed for healthy skin) and magnesium, a lack of which can result in a heart attack. Alcohol is high in calories, serves no useful function nutritionally speaking, and causes the liver to produce acetaldehyde, a toxic cross-linker found in high quantities in drinkers and smokers, which binds proteins together, preventing them from working efficiently, and is thus a prime cause of ageing. Alcohol continues to work invisibly and destructively by clogging tiny blood vessels, interfering with circulation and thus starving the cells of oxygen. As a result, cellular damage and haemorrhages from capillaries that form a network of red veins, acne rosacea, may occur. A glass of dry wine occasionally won't do you any harm, but if you really care about your appearance, it is best to keep 'off the bottle' altogether.

Drugs

Any foreign substance, and all drugs, prescribed or otherwise, come into this category. On entering the bloodstream they are toxic, but are rendered harmless by vitamin C; unfortunately, in defending the body in this way, the vitamin is destroyed.

An editorial in the *Journal of the American Medical Association* entitled 'Is Aspirin a Dangerous Drug?' pointed out that aspirin, which can cause internal haemorrhages, is potentially dangerous if diets contain insufficient vitamin C to detoxify it.

By depleting the body of this valuable anti-ageing vitamin, large doses of which are known to delay the visible signs of ageing, drugs, like cigarettes, actually hasten the process associated with ageing.

PROBLEMS AND SOLUTIONS
Eczema

Research indicates that more and more people are suffering from eczema, a condition that is characterized by an itchy rash and blisters that crust and scale. Eczema of dietary origins and the more stubborn condition known as psoriasis may disappear when biotin (the best source being yeast) and/or linoleic acid (found in lecithin, wheatgerm, seeds and sunflower, safflower, corn and soybean oils) are added to the diet. Eczema around the nose, behind the ears and on the eyebrows and the scalp is one of the most notable symptoms of a B_6 deficiency, a condition that can be corrected by taking 50mg of this vitamin at each meal, in the form of brewer's yeast containing all the B vitamins essential to assimilation. Other sources in descending order are blackstrap molasses, wheatgerm, liver and heart.

Eczema may result from an allergic reaction to such drugs as barbiturates and sulphonamides, or contact with substances like ammonia found in bleaches and household chemicals, lanolin (skin creams and hair preparations), beta-naphthol and ammoniated mercury (freckle creams), barium salts (depilatories), boric acid in lipsticks etc. It is not always easy to identify the allergen, but clues lie in the area where the irritation occurs. If it is the face, check skin creams, lotions and hair preparations; under arms look to depilatories, deodorants and anti-perspirants. Test by smearing a little of the suspect substance on to a plaster and tape it to a freshly washed part of the body. After twenty-four hours remove it. An area showing red irritation indicates that one is allergic to the substance applied to the plaster.

A centuries-old remedy for eczema is to wash the affected area with potato water, made by juicing a raw potato (peeled) in a liquidizer. This helps to cleanse, nourish and heal the skin.

Liver Spots (Lentigines)

Despite their name, so-called 'liver spots' have nothing to do with the liver, but are changes in pigmentation in the skin caused by a prolonged deficiency in certain nutrients, coupled with exposure to sunlight and/or ultraviolet rays from sun lamps.

Vitamin and mineral requirements vary from person to person. Some women, as a result of their genetic make-up, oral contraceptives, extreme stress, and other factors, need a high daily complement of the B vitamins. If the B vitamins, particularly folic acid and (PABA) are insufficient, the greyish-brown pigmentation associated with ageing and other symptoms can occur.

Generally, dermatologists claim that nothing can be done to eliminate these unpleasant discolourations, but a balanced diet supplemented with the B vitamins rich in folic acid and PABA, eliminates them as I have seen. Diet should be improved by taking 16 tablespoons of yogurt (plain) with either one tablespoonful of desiccated liver daily or eating fresh liver once or twice a week. Combine these foods with a good B complex supplement consisting of a minimum of 2mg of folic acid and 300mg of PABA taken with meals, twice a day. This programme, continued indefinitely, will result in clear, lentigines-free skin within six months.

Equally important is to stay out of the sun or at least shield skin by wearing a wide-brimmed hat and cotton gloves. Always avoid sun-screen products that contain oil of bergamot or its derivatives: they have a tendency to accelerate the darkening of the skin even in dull weather, but do not protect the skin from the cellular destruction caused by the sun which results in premature ageing. They are also known to cause allergic reactions in women with allergy-prone, sensitive skins.

AGELESS BEAUTY SKIN CARE PROGRAMME

Dried, Very Wrinkled Skin

A.M.
1 Cleanse by splashing with warm (not hot) water twelve times. Finish with a cool (not cold) water splash twelve times. Do not use soap
2 Either massage the Skin Protector Against Free Radicals into the skin or apply the Cider Vinegar Skin Tonic or any non-alcoholic skin freshener to cotton wool and gently sweep over the skin, taking care to avoid the eyes
3 Apply a rich, day moisturizer lavishly. Using the tips of the fingers, start from the base of the neck using upward strokes, up and over the face
4 Wait a few minutes before applying a second, non-sticky moisturizer of your choice
5 Make-up

P.M.
1 To remove make-up, apply melted cold cream or slightly warm vegetable oil (cold pressed) over the face. Leave for one minute before removing with a clean, wet, warm face flannel. Repeat
2 Cleanse with a rich cleansing cream containing lanolin. Remove with a clean, wet, warm face flannel
3 Cleanse with wheatgerm scrub (optional). (Pour a little wheatgerm in the palm of the hand, moisten with water, and using circular movements, gently massage the skin. Rinse with tepid water)

4   Hydrate the skin. Close eyes and spray with the Glycerine and Mineral Water Hydrator. Repeat several times
5   Pat on eye oil using finger tips. Never rub or pull the skin
6   Apply a night moisturizer of your choice

Additional Treatments
1   Remove dead cells by exfoliating with an oatmeal or an almond scrub once a fortnight
2   Apply warm oil (cold pressed) over the face, and gently massage upwards with the finger tips for five minutes, four times a week
3   Swim or go for a brisk walk in a park or any green, open space for between twenty and thirty minutes three or more times a week

Dried, Slightly Wrinkled Skin

A.M.
1   Wet face thoroughly before cleansing with a non-soap, cleansing foam. Apply with finger tips. Rinse by splashing with tepid water twelve times
2   Either massage the Skin Protector Against Free Radicals into the skin, or apply Cider Vinegar Skin Tonic or any non-alcoholic skin freshener to cotton wool and gently sweep over the skin, taking care to avoid the eyes
3   Apply a day moisturizer lavishly. Using the tips of the fingers, start from the base of the neck using upward strokes, up and over the face
4   Wait a few minutes before applying a second, non-sticky moisturizer of your choice
5   Make-up

P.M.
1   To remove make-up, apply either melted cold cream or slightly warm vegetable oil (cold pressed) over the face. Leave for one minute before removing with a clean, wet, warm face flannel. Repeat
2   Wet face thoroughly before cleansing with a non-soap, cleansing foam. Apply with finger tips. Rinse by splashing with tepid water twelve times
3   Hydrate the skin. Close eyes and spray with the Glycerine and Mineral Water Hydrator. Repeat several times
4   Pat on eye oil using finger tips. Never rub or pull the skin
5   Apply a night moisturizer of your choice

1   Remove dead cells by exfoliating with an oatmeal or an almond scrub once a week
2   Apply warm oil (cold pressed) over the face and gently massage upwards with finger tips for five minutes three times a week
3   Swim or go for a brisk walk in a park or any green, open space for between twenty and thirty minutes three or more times a week

Normal, Very Wrinkled Skin

A.M.
1   Cleanse by splashing with warm (not hot) water thirty times. Finish with a cool (not cold) water splash twelve times. Do not use soap
2   Either massage the Skin Protector Against Free Radicals into the skin or apply either the Cider Vinegar Skin Tonic or any non-alcoholic skin freshener to cotton wool, and gently sweep over the skin taking care to avoid the eyes
3   Apply a nourishing day moisturizer lavishly. Using the tips of the fingers, start from the base of the neck using upward strokes, up and over the face
4   Wait a few minutes before applying a second, non-sticky moisturizer of your choice
5   Make-up

P.M.
1   To remove make-up, apply either melted cold cream or slightly warm vegetable oil (cold pressed) over the face. Leave for one minute before removing with a clean, wet, warm face flannel. Repeat
2   Cleanse with a cream-based cleanser containing lanolin and/or coconut oil. Remove with a clean, wet, warm face flannel
3   Cleanse with wheatgerm scrub (optional)
4   Hydrate the skin. Close the eyes and spray with either the Glycerine and Mineral Water Hydrator or plain mineral water. Repeat several times
5   Pat on eye oil using finger tips. Never rub or pull the skin
6   Apply a night moisturizer of your choice

Additional Treatments
1   Remove dead cells by exfoliating with a sea-salt (fine) scrub once every ten days
2   Apply warm oil (cold pressed) over the face and gently massage upwards with finger tips for five minutes, twice a week
3   Swim or go for a brisk walk in a park or any green, open space for between twenty and thirty minutes three or more times a week

Normal, Slightly Wrinkled Skin

A.M.
1   Wet face thoroughly before cleansing with a non-soap, cleansing foam. Apply with finger tips. Rinse by splashing with cool (not cold) water twelve times
2   Either massage the Skin Protector Against Free Radicals into the skin or apply Cider Vinegar Skin Tonic or any non-alcoholic skin freshener to cotton wool and gently sweep over the skin, taking care to avoid the eyes
3   Apply a day moisturizer lavishly. Using the tips of the fingers, start from the base of the neck using upward strokes, up and over the face
4   Wait a few minutes before applying a second, non-sticky moisturizer of your choice
5   Make-up

P.M.
1   To remove make-up, apply either melted cold cream or slightly warm vegetable oil (cold pressed) over the face. Leave for one minute before removing with a clean, wet, warm face flannel. Repeat
2   Wet face thoroughly before cleansing with a non-soap, cleansing foam. Apply with finger tips. Rinse by splashing with tepid water until no traces remain
3   Hydrate the skin. Close eyes and spray with either the Glycerine and Mineral Water Hydrator or plain mineral water. Repeat several times
4   Pat on eye oil using finger tips. Never rub or pull the skin
5   Apply a night moisturizer of your choice

Additional Treatments
1   Remove dead cells by exfoliating with an oatmeal or an almond scrub once a week
2   Apply warm oil (cold pressed) over the face and gently massage upwards with finger tips for five minutes once a week
3   Swim or go for a brisk walk in a park or any green, open space for between twenty and thirty minutes three or more times a week

Oily, Slightly Wrinkled Skin

A.M.
1   Wet face thoroughly before cleansing with a non-soap cleansing foam. Apply with the finger tips. Rinse by splashing with cool (not cold) water to remove residue

2   Apply an astringent to cotton wool and gently sweep over the avoid the eyes
3   Massage the Skin Protector Against Free Radicals into the skin
4   Apply a day lotion
5   Make-up

P.M.
1   To remove make-up, apply melted cold cream over the face. Leave for one minute before removing with a clean, wet, hot face flannel. Repeat
2   Cleanse with an oatmeal or an almond scrub
3   Hydrate the skin. Close eyes and spray with a solution consisting of equal parts of astringent and mineral water. Repeat
4   Apply a night lotion of your choice

Additional Treatments
1   Remove dead cells by exfoliating with a sea-salt and almond scrub twice a week
2   Apply a deep cleansing mask once a week
3   Swim or go for a brisk walk in a park or any green, open space for between twenty and thirty minutes three or more times a week

A SKINFUL OF BEAUTY

By eating what I call more 'complexion' foods, high in vitamins, minerals and essential trace elements, you are building the foundation of healthy good looks that will last.

However, even with a sensible diet, vitamin and mineral supplements have an important role to play, for they help to augment the nutrients in fresh foods, wholly or partially depleted by the effects of light, air, heat, cooking, handling, storing and freezing.

For a real complexion booster in liquid form, why not try my Iron and Copper Skin Cocktail.

Iron and Copper Skin Cocktail

Put the spinach, parsley and mineral water in a liquidizer and blend until smooth. Add one cup of this rich, dark green liquid to one cup of fresh orange juice and stir thoroughly. Sip slowly. A glassful taken three times a day will do more for your complexion than all the costly toners and blushers on the market.

Another drink which is a superb skin purifier is barley water.

4oz (100 grams) spinach
4oz (100 grams) parsley
1 pint (570ml) mineral water
orange juice (freshly squeezed)

107

Barley Water

4 tablespoonfuls
pearl barley
2 pints (1.15 litres)
water (boiling)
1 lemon (sliced)
1 or 2 oranges
(sliced)
honey to taste

Method 1
Put the washed barley into a jug with the lemon and orange slices and the honey. Add the boiling water, cover and leave to stand for six hours. Strain before use. Refrigerate.

Method 2
This method, which I prefer, requires double the quantity of ingredients. Put the washed barley into a large saucepan, add the boiling water and simmer over a low heat for one hour. Squeeze the juice from the fruits, keeping the juice and the peel separate. Strain the juice into a bowl, add the honey and peel, and leave to stand. When cool, remove the peel and pour in the freshly squeezed fruit juices. Refrigerate.

Natural Skincare Preparations

For years now I have been practising and recommending natural beauty preparations using pure ingredients and the response has been overwhelming. Beauty preparations made at home don't work miracles, but they do work, and extremely effectively too, without allergic reactions and other disadvantages associated with commercial products. Your complexion deserves the best, and skin foods should be nutritionally rich and good enough to eat!

Cider Vinegar Skin Tonic (for Dry and Normal Skins)

2 tablespoonfuls
cider vinegar
16 tablespoonfuls
mineral water

Pour the ingredients into a bottle and replace the lid. Shake vigorously before use. Use this skin tonic to replace the acid mantle after washing.

Skin Protector Against Free Radicals

Pour the four oils into a liquidizer and blend thoroughly. Dissolve the gelatine by adding it to 1 fl oz (35ml) of cold water, then add 3 fl oz (105ml) of boiling water to it, stir and put to one side. When the gelatinous liquid is cool, pour it into the liquidizer together with the remaining ingredients and blend until smooth. Pot, label and refrigerate.

After cleansing, use liberally before applying a moisturizer of your choice.

Note This Skin Protector *must* be used in conjunction with a good moisturizer.

*1 tablespoonful
castor oil
½ tablespoonful
vitamin E oil
½ tablespoonful
almond oil
½ tablespoonful
cod-liver oil
1 tablet (500mg)
vitamin C
(crushed)
1 tablet multi-
vitamin (crushed)
2 tablespoonfuls
orange juice
(freshly squeezed)
½ tablespoonful
gelatine*

Glycerine and Mineral Water Hydrator

Pour the ingredients into a new and clean plant 'mister', and replace the lid. Shake vigorously before spraying over the skin. Pat almost but not quite dry. Repeat throughout the day whenever possible.

*3 teaspoonfuls
glycerine
1 pint (570ml)
mineral water*

Nourishing Night Cream for Mature Skins

Melt the honey in a small saucepan over a low heat, and put to one side. When cool, add the egg yolks, cream and oil and whisk until smooth and creamy. Pot up, label and refrigerate. Apply lavishly to face and neck.

*1 small carton
double cream
3 teaspoonfuls
honey
1 teaspoonful
wheatgerm oil
2 egg yolks*

Mayonnaise Revitalizing Cream

12 tablespoonfuls safflower oil
2 tablespoonfuls cider vinegar
1 teaspoonful honey
1 teaspoonful sea salt (fine)
1 egg yolk

Place the egg yolk, one-third of the oil and one-quarter teaspoonful of sea salt into a bowl or a liquidizer and blend thoroughly. Pour in another one-third of the oil and mix well before finally adding the vinegar, honey and the remaining ingredients. Blend until smooth. Pot up, label and refrigerate.

Apply this cream after washing in the morning and continue to apply it as often as possible throughout the day. You will notice a considerable improvement within a matter of weeks.

EXERCISE – THE NATURAL FACE LIFT

Sagging neck and facial muscles that alter the overall symmetry of the face is an aspect of ageing that women dread the most. The face requires and deserves the daily care of the Ageless Beauty Skin Care Programme, but it also needs something more: regular exercise. Like the body, the face is a sculpture of muscles that need regular work-outs to maintain firm muscles and youthful contours, but unlike work-outs in a gym, far less time and effort is needed to strengthen, firm and tone facial muscles and smooth out wrinkles. Facial exercises done regularly re-model an ageing, drooping face to younger, more rounded contours, and as muscles in the face become stronger and circulation tones up, one's natural skin colour also improves. Whatever one's age, it is never too late to give one's face a lift.

Once you have mastered these simple exercises, you can do them whenever you are alone, either taking a bath (this is the best time of all), or doing housework, or preparing a meal or watching television. It is simply a matter of including them in your daily routine. Facial exercises must be done with cold-pressed oil or a rich, moisturizing cream. Lifting the face without lubricating the skin first may deepen rather than smooth out existing wrinkles.

When trying these facially rejuvenating exercises for the first time, sit in front of a mirror to check that you are doing them correctly. Try to concentrate on the individual muscles you are working and the beneficial effects the exercise is having.

Facial Exercises

Exercise 1
Known as the 'Lion', this exercise stretches and tones muscles and improves circulation to the face, neck and larynx. However, it should only be done when you are alone for reasons that become clear.

Sit on an upright chair so that your head and back are straight. Open your eyes and mouth wide and extend your tongue down towards your chin as far as possible, with great force. Hold for six seconds, relax and repeat a minimum of six times.

Exercise 2
For those who want to counteract sagging, drooping, flabby muscles, this facial 'up-lifter' is the one for you.

Sit in front of a mirror with your chin protruding very slightly. Now with your mouth half-open, smile upwards as hard as possible so that your face and neck muscles are pulled tight into this smiling position. Hold for twenty seconds, relax and repeat.

Exercise 3
Among the numerous exercises for stimulating the entire face at once, this one called 'Happy Face' is a favourite of mine. To enjoy the full benefit of this exercise, you need to feel happy and fairly relaxed, so get yourself in the mood and release your inhibitions by opening your eyes and mouth as wide as possible. That's it, stretch so that your face has a wide-eyed, open-mouthed look of joyous surprise. Doesn't it make you feel good?

Now comes the exercise. Keeping your mouth closed, grit your back teeth, hold for ten seconds, relax and repeat.

Exercise 4
Fill your mouth with air so that your mouth and cheeks are puffed out. Now, roll the air around inside your mouth, as if you are trying to chew a mouthful of food with difficulty. Hold for twenty seconds before releasing the air suddenly with a pop! Repeat.

Exercise 5
This eye exercise reduces frown lines on the forehead, smooths out the tiny wrinkles on or near the eyelids and between the eyebrows, and helps prevent sagging immediately below the eyes.

Having oiled the entire face, concentrating particularly on the area around the eyes, close one eye hard and lift and tense the entire face on the same side into a wink and a smile. Hold for one second, relax and repeat thirty times each side.

Exercise 6
This face lift is designed to smooth out crease lines between the nose and the upper lip.

Place your thumbs just above the top lip and push upwards towards your nose as your lip muscles pull downwards to resist the upward pull. Hold for six seconds, relax and repeat.

Exercise 7
An excellent work out for exercising and toning chin and jaw muscles.

Put out your tongue and try and touch your nose. Hold for six seconds and repeat.

Exercise 8
This exercise is wonderful for preventing a double chin. It is not easy to do at first, but persevere until you get it right. Put your hands together and clasp your fingers tightly. Now push your interlocked hands against your chin, whilst at the same time pushing your chin against your hands. Hold the pressure for twenty seconds, relax and repeat. Keep trying for it is well worth the effort.

Exercise 9
A tightener that helps to keep chin and neck firm and line-free.

Open your mouth an inch, no more, widen it into a broad smile and bite down hard on an imaginary apple. Hold for six seconds and repeat. Can't you feel the muscles responding?

Exercise 10
Good for toning and maintaining the youthful contours of the neck.

Sit with your head and shoulders straight. Without moving your head, draw down the corners of your mouth into a grimace. Hold for six seconds, relax and repeat.

Exercise 11
For this neck-lift, imagine that your chin is supporting a small but very heavy box, which you are trying to lift up. Raise your chin upwards and contract the muscles underneath enough to maintain that heavy weight. Hold for six seconds, relax and repeat a minimum of six times.

Exercise 12
For this neck tightener, sit on a hard-backed chair so that your back is upright and your shoulders straight. Now, bend your head over to one side so that your ear is almost touching your shoulder – don't try to raise your shoulder to your ear, that's cheating! Hold for ten seconds, relax and repeat on the other side. Done correctly, you will feel all the neck muscles, ones you have hardly used, coming into play.

7
Eyes

EYE NUTRITION

The eyes 'mirror the soul' and 'light up' the personality, but what they reflect more accurately still is lifestyle and general health. A doctor examining the eyes with the aid of a thin pencil of light can recognize and diagnose ailments that affect not just the eye itself but the brain and other parts of the body suffering from brain tumours, diabetes, leukaemia, atherosclerosis and kidney disease. Bright eyes that have a bluish tinge to the white and really sparkle denote vitality of a kind that can only be achieved by health that is based on sound nutrition. In fact, one only has to see how nutritional deficiencies adversely affect the eyes to realize the importance of good foods and their absorption and utilization.

A lack of vitamins A, B_2, B_6, inositol, C, E, and the amino acids that make up proteins are responsible for a host of eye abnormalities. A good example is vitamin A, a deficiency of which, even a slight one, can cause impaired vision, particularly 'night blindness' which makes it difficult to see in the dark, and tests have shown that motorists involved in accidents after dark are often lacking this vitamin. Other symptoms include a sensitivity to bright light, and typists and office workers who face the glare of light on white paper and skiers and mountain climbers exposed to the reflection of sun on newly fallen snow are particularly susceptible to eyestrain and visual difficulties. If the deficiency worsens, burning, itching and inflamed eyelids are experienced.

Sensitivity to bright light and faulty vision in poor, dimmed light are early symptoms of a B_2 deficiency. Unlike people deficient in vitamin A, night vision remains normal, provided the diet is adequate in all other nutrients. If the condition continues and worsens, the sufferer experiences watering eyes, burning, itchy eyelids and possibly even splitting of the skin at the outer corners of the eyes. Bloodshot eyes and cataracts occur in people lacking B_6 and certain amino acids.

Inositol, a member of the B complex group, is normally concentrated in the lens of the human eye, which seems to indicate that one of its tasks is in maintaining healthy vision. Laboratory animals fed on a diet lacking this vitamin develop eye abnormalities of various kinds, among other symptoms.

Vitamin C also plays a major role in maintaining normal vision. Like inositol, it too, is concentrated in the lenses of healthy eyes, but people with cataracts of certain types are found to be low or lacking in this important vitamin. Improvements in eye infections can be expected after massive doses of vitamin C have been given, whereas a restricted vitamin C intake has actually produced experimental cataracts, so confirming its role in maintaining visual health.

Vitamin E has been used successfully in the treatment of various eye disorders. Premature babies become blind if they are placed in oxygen tents where the pressure is so high that it causes retrolental fibroplasia, an eye disorder that is responsible for more blindness in babies than any other condition. However, in one study a group of these infants were given vitamin E daily, starting immediately after birth, and retained their sight whereas over one-fifth of those untreated turned blind. Children that are cross-eyed may also have been treated successfully with vitamin E, which strengthens the eye muscles and so helps to correct the condition. Dosage varies from person to person and should be administered only under careful medical supervision. Although vitamin E and its role in eye health is well established, it is still ignored by all but those members of the medical profession with a nutritional approach to treatment.

PROBLEMS AND SOLUTIONS

Swollen, Puffy Eyes

Lack of sleep is normally responsible for red and puffy eyes. I admire women who look and function their best on four or five hours' sleep a night, but a good night's sleep for me is eight hours. If necessary, I can function fairly well on seven hours but less than seven or more than eight hours a night, and I am little more than an automaton. Research at the State Health Department in California shows that to live longer and stay healthier,

114

and this is the aim of us all, one needs a minimum of seven hours but not more than eight hours per night.

Only during sleep can eyes really rest. Other common causes of swollen eyes are inadequate diet and a constipated, 'clogged-up' system. Water is a wonderful internal cleanser and one's day should always begin with a large glass of tepid mineral water. Swollen, irritated eyes might be a reaction to heavy creams applied lavishly to the surrounding eyes at night. A good eye cream glides on easily and should be tapped lightly in using the third finger. Never rub, tug or pull the skin. Finish by blotting any surplus cream with a tissue prior to retiring.

If having taken these precautions under-eye puffiness still occurs, try one of the following natural cures. For centuries, raw potato has been used to alleviate swollen lids. The quickest way is to place a slice of peeled, raw potato on each eye. Alternatively, cover each with a doubled square of gauze or muslin containing grated, raw potato. Lie back with your eyes closed for fifteen minutes before rinsing with cool water. Cotton wool dipped in chamomile or eyebright 'tea', applied to the eyes every five minutes, each time using freshly soaked pads, also relieves red and inflamed eyes. Chamomile tea should be brewed in the normal way and left to stand for twenty minutes before straining ready for use. Eyebright tea is made by infusing two tablespoons of the dried herb in two cups of hot water. Allow to cool before use.

Blurred Vision and Tired Eyes

The strain of reading or writing in poor light for long periods manifests itself as blurred vision and dull, bloodshot eyes. Fortunately, I have excellent sight, yet a few years ago working for hours on end without a break was affecting my vision to such a degree that, when out walking, everything looked blurred. Friends suggested that I probably needed glasses, bifocals generally being regarded as an instant remedy for failing sight, but I realized that glasses were not the solution. My sight was suffering because my eyes were being subjected to close work over long periods. Since then, I regularly rest them by either focusing on an object at the farthest end of the room, or better still, sitting by an upstairs window and concentrating on a distant landmark, an exercise which, I find, both relaxes and strengthens my eyes.

Not an exercise so much as a tonic for tired eyes, and one to which I always resort after a tiring day, is 'palming'. As the name implies, the palms of the hands are placed over closed eyes and pressed gently against them for two minutes. Meanwhile, relax your body and breathe slowly and deeply to refresh the rest of you.

If eyes become tired easily, unnaturally so, after reading or watching television for example, particularly if accompanied by headaches and sensitivity to bright light, and there seems no logical reason, a lack of vitamin A could be responsible. Try to include more vitamin A-rich foods in your diet. Good sources are liver, carrots, tomatoes, kale, spinach, broccoli, cabbage and other green vegetables.

Dark Circles

I don't need to tell you how lack of sleep and stress affects your looks, especially your eyes. Yet, even with adequate sleep and a relaxed lifestyle, you may still have dark rims below the eyes. Two factors that are likely to be responsible are anaemia and poor elimination. The Internal Cleansing Plan to cleanse the system of impurities followed by either the Stress-Reducing Menu or the Weight-Reducing Ageless Beauty Diet usually eradicates them within a matter of weeks. However, if you enjoy your present diet and don't wish to change your eating habits, the High-Fibre Start to the Day will provide you with the sort of breakfast that encourages elimination. Afterwards and throughout the day, try to avoid foods high in carbohydrates and low in antacid such as white bread, pastries, white flour products and pasta dishes etc., all of which when digested release high levels of acid and carbon dioxide gas, which makes blood look darker than usual, and thus show through the fine skin below the eyes. Eat more fresh green and yellow vegetables and plenty of fruits, especially oranges, tangerines, pineapples and grapefruits. I have never suffered from 'panda eyes', but I learned from a reliable source who does that papaya mint tea brewed and applied to the eyes in the same way as chamomile tea (see page 89) helps alleviate the problem.

Eye Lines and Wrinkles

In contrast to the fatty tissue on the body, the eyelids and the fine, delicate skin surrounding the eyes, have no oil glands, and therefore need to be kept well lubricated at all times. I have tried oils of various kinds and find that castor oil helps to keep the skin moist and supple – it is also a very efficient eye make-up remover – but for real results, try vitamin E oil. After cleansing, puncture a 200iu vitamin E capsule with a pin and apply under the eyes, repeating throughout the day and before retiring at night, when the upper lids can be treated too.

For that special occasion when you want to look your best but don't know how to make those tiny lines below the eyes less noticeable, use the Anti-Line Eye Preparation on page 118. Another recipe with marvellous skin-tightening properties is the Honey Under-Eye Treatment, also on page 118.

As mentioned in Chapter 6, there is a definite correlation between 'crow's feet' and smoking, so if you are alarmed by the 'feet' on your face, make an effort to break this unhealthy and unbeautiful habit once and for all.

EYE EXERCISES

All these exercises help to strengthen eyes and improve vision.

Exercise 1
Sit on an upright chair placed against a wall, half-way into the room, and rest your head against the wall. Keeping your head quite still, focus on a corner of the ceiling, and slowly move your eyes from that corner to the opposite one and back again. Repeat several times.

Exercise 2
Imagine you are watching a game of tennis. Using your eyes, not your neck, follow the ball left right, right left, left right.

Exercise 3
Imagine that you are looking at a large clock face. Again using only your eye muscles, focus on number 12 and then move down to 6. Now move from 1 to 7; 2 to 8; 3 to 9; 4 to 10; 5 to 11; 6 to 12; 7 to 1; 8 to 2; 9 to 3; 10 to 4; 11 to 5; and 12 to 6. Now repeat in an anti-clockwise direction: 12 to 6; 11 to 5; 10 to 4; 9 to 3; 8 to 2; 7 to 1; 6 to 12; 5 to 11; 4 to 10; 3 to 9; 2 to 8; 1 to 7 and 12 to 6.

Exercise 4
Still focusing on the clock, start at 6 and slowly move to 7; 8; 9; 10; 11; 12; 1; 2; 3; 4; 5 and 6. Now repeat in an anti-clockwise direction, starting at 6 and moving to 5; 4; 3; 2; 1; 12; 11; 10; 9; 8; 7 and 6.

SPECIAL EYE TREATMENTS

Anti-Line Eye Preparation

1 egg white
mineral water (non-carbonated)

Mix the egg white and about half as much mineral water. Using a small artist's brush, brush the preparation across the area under the eyes. When dry, apply foundation or base make-up over it. As the skin tightens, so it will smooth out the lines, but sadly, the effect is only a temporary one.

Honey Under-Eye Treatment

1 egg white
1 teaspoon honey

Blend the ingredients together. Pot up, label and refrigerate. Dab this mixture below the eyes and gently pat it in. When thoroughly dry, rinse off with tepid water, pat dry, and apply a good eye oil. This treatment helps to iron out lines and wrinkles.

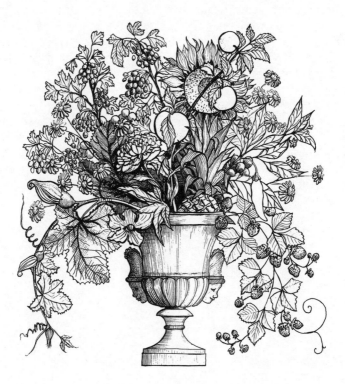

8
Hair

HAIR NUTRITION

Heredity has a lot to do with good hair, but bad eating habits and incorrect care, not genetic factors, are to blame for thin, lifeless hair that lacks body and lustre.

Like skin, hair also needs feeding from within with good quality foods and many basic hair problems can be corrected by replacing the 'non-food' fillers like sweets, cakes, pastries, biscuits, chocolate, soft drinks, sugar etc., with first-class proteins. The basic need for protein, not too much, but enough to supply the body without depleting it of the minerals it needs, is understandable, for hair consists of 98 per cent protein. By following the Weight-Reducing Ageless Beauty Diet or the Stress-Reducing Menu, whichever is more suitable, will ensure healthy, all-over beauty that will withstand the test of time. In addition, supplements to strengthen and promote hair growth and help prevent premature greying should be taken daily until the condition of the hair has improved.

Vitamin A

Vitamin A is considered an important skin nutrient but it is essential to hair health as well. An undersupply can cause hair to become dry, dull and fall out in extreme cases and these symptoms are likely to be accompanied by an accumulation of dandruff. A well-balanced diet will ensure an adequate supply, but more foods rich in this vitamin can be included, if necessary, without risk of toxicity. Another way to ensure that intake is commensurate with individual requirements, and this can vary from person to person, is to take cod-liver oil as a supplement (see page 15).

The B Vitamins

The B vitamins are the key to beautiful hair, for they strengthen the hair shaft and promote luxuriant growth. One of the B vitamins, namely para-aminobenzoic acid (PABA) is known as the anti-grey hair vitamin because animals lacking it turn grey, but biotin, folic acid, and pantothenic acid also affect hair colour. A reversal of the greying process has been achieved under medical supervision, by prescribing supplements of these vitamins in mega-doses. Animals deprived of biotin and inositol exhibit various symptoms including loss of hair and these, together with choline, appear to be responsible for hair growth.

Dr Benjamin Sieve of Boston, Massachusetts, prescribed PABA to three hundred patients with grey hair whose ages ranged from sixteen to seventy-four and changes in hair colour occurred within five weeks of treatment. Patients formerly blonde developed a yellowish, somewhat muddy colour initially, which gradually changed to their original hair colour. Others, formerly brunettes, turned dark grey before assuming their normal shade of brown. The overall condition of the hair also improved. The daily dose consisted of 100mg of PABA (divided into small doses that were taken between two and six times with meals throughout the day). For premature greying, Dr Sieve prescribed 50mg daily (until the yellow or grey stage is reached), thereafter increasing to 100mg daily (divided into small, daily doses as recommended above).

Here is a formula designed to prevent hair turning grey.

Anti-Grey Hair Formula

2,000mg (2 grams) choline
   30mg PABA
   30mg calcium pantothenate

Note: Do not take PABA or any one B vitamin by itself, because it increases the need for the remaining Bs that are absent. The doses recommended must be taken as part of a B complex formula containing all the B vitamins.

For habitual tea and coffee drinkers, the outlook is truly grey! These liquids taken in large quantities daily can result in a depletion of the water-soluble B vitamins from the system and the B deficiency that results can cause premature greying of the hair.

Vitamin C

Vitamin C helps rebuild tissues including those of the hair and the skin, detoxifies the blood and maintains healthy capillaries through which nutrients are directed to the hair follicles. An undersupply results in haemorrhaging of the capillary walls which, in turn, impedes nourishment to the papillae. As stated in Chapter 6, stress, tobacco, alcohol, aspirin and other drugs are all depleters of vitamin C. For more information, turn to the vitamin chart on page 39.

Copper

Animals lacking this trace element show typical symptoms of anaemia and this may be accompanied by greying and loss of hair. Copper deficiency is not easily recognized in the human animal, but a deficiency of copper, or indeed any mineral, is likely to show up in the hair before it is apparent elsewhere. Good sources of copper are liver, brains and kidneys, but these foods are not popular with everyone. Alternatively, a good multi-vitamin and mineral tablet containing copper and other trace elements is recommended.

Iron

A mineral of primary importance in maintaining healthy hair growth is iron. The hair of anaemic women lacks lustre, is difficult to manage and tends to break easily. If an iron deficiency is suspected, symptoms of which are described in the mineral chart on page 52, make an appointment with your doctor and ask for a serum iron test. If, as a result, an iron supplement is prescribed, remember to take it with vitamin C and a glass of milk, both of which improve iron absorption. Women who are prematurely grey or in extreme cases, have partially lost their hair due to an iron deficiency, or a lack of pantothenic acid, or other B vitamins over a prolonged period, have been helped by taking one teaspoonful of blackstrap molasses in a glass of milk, daily.

Sulphur

Known as Nature's 'beauty mineral', sulphur is a constituent of keratin of which the innermost layer of the hair shaft is composed. Good natural sources and supplements are discussed in the Mineral and Trace Element Chart on page 52.

Zinc

Zinc is important to strong hair and luxuriant growth, and is believed to prevent hair loss to some extent. Research indicates that both animals and humans with a severe zinc deficiency develop similar symptoms, which include skin abnormalities, particularly psoriasis, a scalp condition that can spread to other parts of the body and is difficult to treat. Like the water-soluble B vitamins, zinc is also excreted in the urine if too much liquid is consumed or diuretics taken.

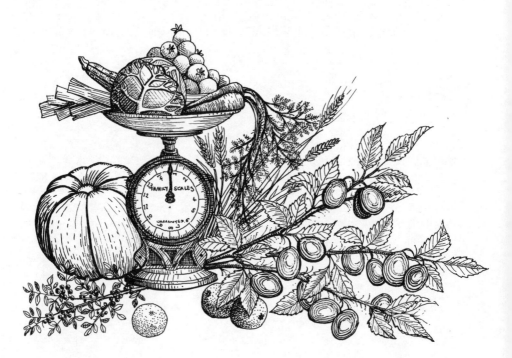

Anita Guyton's Healthy Hair Cocktail

Place all the ingredients in a liquidizer and blend until smooth. Drink one cupful in the morning, a second one mid-day and a third in the evening. You will notice an improvement in your hair within a matter of months.

Note: If hair is very dry increase the quantity of olive oil.

1½ pints (850ml) milk (skimmed)
8 tablespoons yogurt (plain)
¼ pint (140ml) cucumber juice (fresh)
1 large banana or a handful of strawberries if in season
2 eggs
2 tablespoons brewer's yeast (powder)
2 tablespoons wheatgerm flakes
2 tablespoons dried, powdered milk
1 tablespoon wheatgerm oil
1 tablespoon lecithin
2 teaspoons olive oil (virgin)
6 desiccated-liver tablets (crushed)
2 multi-vitamin and mineral tablets (crushed)
1,000mg vitamin C

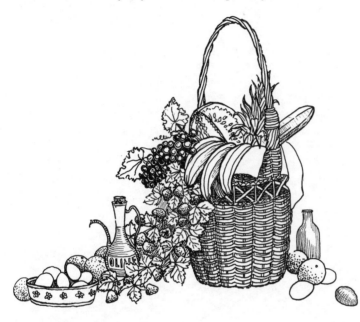

Anti-Grey Hair Cocktail

Place all the ingredients in a liquidizer and blend until smooth. Take one glassful three times a day.

Try to keep your intake of tea, coffee and alcohol to a minimum and take two of the three glasses of this Anti-Grey Hair Cocktail last thing at night before retiring to help ensure minimum excretion and maximum absorption (remember to brush your teeth afterwards!)

The consistency of this cocktail can vary, depending on the yogurt used. Homemade yogurt (see page 25) is nutritionally superior to commercial brands and the consistency makes it ideal for this recipe.

1½ pints (850ml) milk (skimmed)
3 tablespoons brewer's yeast (powder)
3 tablespoons wheatgerm
2 tablespoons blackstrap molasses
16 tablespoons yogurt (plain)

DIETARY DOS AND DON'TS

A correct diet is a significant part of healthy hair. Following the Weight-Reducing Ageless Beauty Diet or the Stress-Reducing Menu and supplementing it with nutrients essential for health and hair beauty will contribute enormously to the overall improvement of the hair. Of course, if you do not wish to completely revise your eating habits but nevertheless still wish to improve the condition of your hair, here is a list of the dietary do's and don'ts.

Do
- Try to eat small quantities of first-class protein (lean meat, liver, fish, chicken etc.) once a day
- Eat an egg three times a week
- Try to have one green salad at least once a day
- Eat fresh vegetables (consisting of at least one green, leafy one), preferably raw, daily. If you feel that you must have cooked vegetables, lightly steam but never overcook them or all the nutrients will be lost
- Nibble on fresh fruit, a minimum of two pieces, one of which is an orange, daily
- Take vitamin and mineral supplements immediately after eating
- Drink a minimum of six glasses of mineral water instead of tea, coffee or alcohol, daily if your diet is high in carbohydrate/low in raw fruit and vegetables

Don't
- Eat fried foods; they are hair and skin killers. Grilling, poaching or steaming is kinder to hair and waistline
- Eat 'junk', processed or prepared meals or tinned meats, fruits or vegetables, all of which are low in vitamins and minerals, high in carbohydrates and loaded with salt, sugar and fats
- Indulge (except occasionally) in cheeses with a high fat content (Cheddar, Swiss, American Blue, Roquefort, Camembert and full fat cream cheeses are high in fat). Turn to mozzarella, cottage and low-fat soft cheeses
- Buy white bread. Change to granary or wholegrain bread
- Eat butter. Try polyunsaturated margarine instead or soya bean butter
- Drink whole (full fat) milk. Skimmed or semi-skimmed has more calcium, less fat and fewer calories
- Eat cream except on special occasions. Try yogurt or soya cream (see page 18) or milk sweetened with a little honey over fresh fruit salad
- Use salt. All the salt needed by the body is in the foods we eat
- Add sugar. Instead use honey or blackstrap molasses as a sweetener
- Eat sweets, cakes, pastries, biscuits, chocolate etc., which are bad for hair, skin and waistline.

SCALP MASSAGE

The damage stress can do to health is well known, but its effect on hair is no less dramatic and just as traumatic.

Stress over a prolonged period, characterized by feelings of tightness across the shoulders, up the neck and into the scalp, known as 'tight scalp syndrome', causes the arrector pili muscles, where the hair grows out of the scalp, to contract and the reduced flow of blood and oxygen that results can cause hair loss. In addition, secretions of sweat combined with dust etc., make the scalp and hair dirtier and the sebaceous glands' increased oil secretions result in heavier dandruff.

Scalp massage won't stop balding in men, nor will it prevent the normal loss, usually of between one and two hundred hairs a day, but this daily exercise will stimulate the flow of blood to the scalp, thus increasing the oxygen and nutrient supplies to the hair follicles which, in turn, improves hair growth considerably.

Scalp massage and its effects were obvious to me from a very early age. My grandmother had the habit of kneading the base of her scalp with her fingertips when she was preoccupied. As she moved from her fifties into her sixties, her hair turned iron-grey, but the massaged section remained black to the day she died, which, on reflection, could only have been due to this stimulation.

I cannot promise that daily massage is the panacea for greying hair but it certainly will ease a taut scalp, produce stronger hair growth and promote relaxation and a general feeling of well-being.

Bending the head forward, slide the fingers through the hair on to the scalp, and using the soft pads, not the nails, knead in a series of circular movements, moving the scalp, not the fingers. Work in one position for about one minute before moving on to the next spot and so on, until you have exercised the whole scalp. Always work from the hairline to the sides and over the crown to the base of the neck; the same direction as the blood flows to reach the heart. Done carefully, massage makes the scalp tingle and feel warm and loose. Combine it with the Slant-Board Relaxer for optimum results.

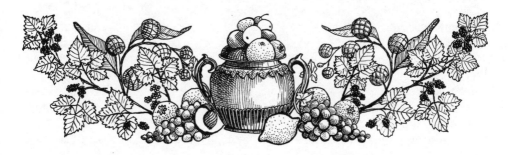

PROBLEMS AND SOLUTIONS

Dry Hair

Dry hair looks dull, tangles quickly, is generally coarse and frizzy and breaks easily due to a loss of elasticity. Hair in peak condition has excellent elasticity and will stretch an average 25 per cent, and as much as 35 per cent of its length before breaking. Test hair for dryness by taking a hair, laying it along a ruler, stretching it between your fingers and measuring how far it stretches before it snaps. If the elasticity is less than 25 per cent of the length, you almost certainly have dry hair and the problems associated with it.

Common causes of dry hair are a) a lack of sebum from the hair follicles and b) a loss of moisture from the hair shaft. The former can be corrected by replenishing the oils in your system by incorporating polyunsaturated, cold-pressed vegetable oils in the diet, and supplementing them, if necessary, with cod-liver oil.

Bleaching and colouring and outdoor sports like golf, tennis and swimming etc., where hair is subjected to constant sun, wind and water are responsible for moisture loss from the hair shaft that results in dryness. Such activities are excellent ways of staying fit and should continue but protect your hair with a hat or a bathing cap.

Once you begin to a) improve your diet, b) cut down or better still eliminate salt altogether, c) include cold-pressed vegetable oils and cod-liver oil in the daily diet and d) take precautionary measures to minimize sun, wind and water damage, additional treatments to combat dry hair should be considered.

Dry Hair Treatment

Dry hair needs to be shampooed and conditioned frequently, but it is fragile and needs delicate treatment. When buying a shampoo, select a thin, fairly liquid one with as few additives, such as proteins, emollients, conditioners etc., as possible. Such a shampoo is likely to have a higher concentration of active ingredients and therefore cleans more efficiently in smaller quantities. Furthermore, diluting shampoo by adding distilled water actually improves its overall performance. The way in which a conditioner is used will determine the final result as much as the ingredients it contains, but more about shampoos and conditioners later.

In addition to shampooing and conditioning, dry hair needs a warm oil treatment once or twice a week if hair is extremely dry, and particularly during the summer months. Take between a quarter and a half cup of corn, olive, almond, or sunflower oil or any good-quality cold-pressed vegetable oil (the quantity depending on the length of the

126

hair), and heat to a pleasant warmness. Now, part the hair down the middle and apply oil liberally and evenly beginning at the roots and working down to the ends. Part the hair again about one inch away and repeat the process. When every strand is oiled, comb the hair thoroughly to ensure even distribution. Next, dip your finger tips in the oil remaining and using finger tips, not nails, massage the scalp for between five and seven minutes. Following the massage, place a plastic bag over the head and envelop in a warm towel. Leave for a minimum of thirty minutes, but if the minutes turn into hours, so much the better.

Grey Hair

Medical nutritionists in the USA, who have carried out research into the anti-grey hair vitamins, are convinced that grey hair signifies a nutritional deficiency and is not, as is generally believed, a natural consequence of ageing.

Many experts in the field of nutrition and beauty report numerous cases where grey hair has returned to its original colour through nutrition alone. Research has established that a pantothenic acid deficiency causes premature greying of the hair in laboratory animals, but restoration of the vitamin to the diet re-colours the hair. Adelle Davis, the doyen of nutritionists, is quoted in *Secrets of Health and Beauty* by Linda Clark, as saying:

'Probably every nutrient influences the health of the hair.

'Adequate amounts of iron, copper, iodine, and the following B vitamins are essential in maintaining the natural colour of the hair: pantothenic acid (calcium pantothenate), PABA, folic acid, and inositol. Grey hair at any age, particularly prematurely grey hair, probably indicates a deficiency of one or more of these nutrients.

'The natural colour of grey hair has sometimes been restored by an adequate intake of all the anti-grey hair vitamins. The most marked results in restoration of colour of grey hair have come from a liberal use of natural foods supplying B vitamins, brewer's yeast, blackstrap molasses, wheatgerm, rice polishings, liver and yogurt.

'When liberal amounts of yogurt are taken daily, the yogurt bacteria growing in the intestinal tract apparently synthesize or produce the B vitamins inositol, and other anti-grey hair vitamins. The richest sources of inositol are whole wheat breads, brewer's yeast, blackstrap molasses and wheatgerm.'

For more information on these vitamins and natural foods, turn to Hair Nutrition (page 119), the Vitamin Chart (page 39), The Wonder Foods (page 13), and the Anti-Grey Hair Cocktail (page 123).

Other established causes of greying hair are heredity, anaemia, inadequate copper, iron and iodine, undernourished glands, stress and poor circulation of the scalp.

Of these, heredity is a major consideration. That is to say, if either your mother or your father were completely grey at the age of forty-five, the probability is that you too will turn grey at that age, but because greying is also associated with other factors, it is by no means inevitable.

Anaemia and the problems that arise from nutritional deficiencies can be corrected by dietary improvements and vitamin and mineral supplements. Uncontrolled stress, and its potential dangers, can also be alleviated in a number of ways as shown in Chapter 5. Poor scalp circulation can be stimulated into increased activity by scalp massage (see page 125) and regular use of the Slant-Board Relaxer (see page 91), both of which should become part of one's daily routine. Scalp circulation can be boosted still further by taking vitamin E each day. Start with 100 units daily and gradually increase the dosage to between 400 and 600iu daily, as recommended in the Vitamin Chart.

Certainly hair colouring the nutritional way and the exercises designed to stimulate scalp circulation and generally improve hair health are worth trying. The heads of many people are testimony to their effectiveness. I hope that you too, will be among them.

Falling and Thinning Hair

A head of healthy hair usually consists of between 90,000 and 140,000 hair follicles, each containing a hair. Redheads have the least number of hairs (about 90,000) followed by black with approximately 110,000, brunettes nearer 120,000 and blondes who have approximately 140,000 or so, although it doesn't actually look thicker because the hairs tend to be finer.

Hair develops in three phases; the growing or the anagen phase; the resting (the catagen stage) which lasts only a matter of weeks, and the falling or the telogen period when it reaches the end of its cycle and is dislodged by a younger, more vibrant hair. The lifespan of each hair varies from between two to five years, depending on the health and genetic make-up of the individual, which means that an entire head of hair is replaced over a five-year period.

In the normal course of events, we can expect to lose between twenty and one hundred hairs per day without even noticing it, and in the same way animals shed their coats seasonally, we too tend to lose noticeably more hairs in the late autumn and early spring.

Excessive hair loss – and by 'excessive' I mean handfuls at a time – can have a variety of causes. During pregnancy, after the birth of the baby, and around the time of menopause, due to a hormonal imbalance, during periods of stress and the 'tight scalp' syndrome that generally accompanies them, and prolonged periods of poor nutrition that result in anaemia, are specific times in a woman's life when excessive hair shedding is most likely.

Vitamin A is involved in the growth and repair of the body and its role is vital to health, but intakes in excess of bodily requirements can cause hair to fall out. People who buy self-prescribed vitamin A seem to be unaware that mega-doses in tablet or capsule form daily, as opposed to natural sources which are quite safe, regardless of dosage, can be retained in the body and a continual build-up might prove toxic. If the diet includes plenty of fresh foods rich in this vitamin, and is supplemented with fish-liver oil or capsules daily, further vitamin A is ordinarily neither necessary nor desirable.

Illnesses like influenza, typhoid and other fevers and treatments of diseases that involve cortisone such as those of multiple sclerosis and chemotherapy in the case of cancer, can cause hair loss in varying degrees, which though distressing is reversible. Other prescribed drugs, for example sedatives, diet pills and the 'Pill' for birth control, and drugs for so-called 'recreational' purposes like marijuana or amphetamines (and here the list is endless), can damage health in general and hair in particular, resulting in excessive hair shedding. Even aspirin, which is considered innocuous, though mistakenly so in my opinion, taken too liberally, has been known to result in hair loss. If hair falls out within a month or two after taking a drug, prescribed or otherwise, seek help without delay.

Other common causes of hair loss, thinning or breaking are maltreatments using stiff nylon brushes, rollers, driers, perms, bleaches and straightening agents and cornrows, tight plaits, ponytails and other hairstyles that put great pressure on hair and cause traction alopecia.

I know how alarming it is when hair comes out in handfuls, having suffered it myself, but try not to worry because it will only make matters worse. Instead, try to discover the cause(s) by a process of elimination and then take the steps necessary to correct the condition, which may include consultations with either a doctor, a trichologist or a drug dependency unit.

Split Ends

Hair that 'forks' at the tips is a minor disorder which occurs when the individual cell layers separate in the oldest part of the hair, namely the ends, as a result of poor hair care. The Latin name, scissura pilorum, is a term that is used to clients to impress the seriousness of the condition, the implication being that immediate treatment is called for. This suggestion is ridiculous and somewhat akin to singeing the hair to seal the hollow shaft and thus prevent life-giving 'energy' from escaping from the hair, an equally outmoded idea borne of ignorance. Equally contrary to popular belief is the fact that protein conditioners are incapable of bonding the split ends together. The only remedy is to cut off the split ends and prevent their re-occurrence by treating hair unhurriedly and with kindness. Never use sharp-edged or broken combs and brushes, or brushes with nylon bristles, which could snag and damage hair. When brushing hair, particularly if it is long, use slow, gentle, even strokes to minimize pressure on the ends. Avoid sun damage, chlorinated swimming pools and shampoos that are extremely alkaline, and be sparing with hair treatments that involve bleaches, electric hair curlers and blow driers. If you can't do without heated curlers – frequent use can cause split ends – protect the hair by wrapping the ends in tissue paper before applying the heated rollers.

Dandruff

Few of us admit to dandruff without experiencing feelings of acute embarrassment, but this disorder can be a health problem, and as such should be regarded in the same way as a cold or a bout of flu.

A term used to describe all flaking and scaling conditions of the scalp, dandruff can spread to any area of the skin where the sebaceous glands are most numerous. Known as the seborrhoeaic areas, they include the scalp, the corners of the eyebrows, along the sides of the nose near the cheeks, the chin, the back, the chest, and occasionally the arms and legs.

Dandruff appears in many forms, from common dandruff that itches and when scratched falls away easily, to psoriasis, a more difficult disorder where the scales, silver-white in colour, cling tenaciously to the scalp, and neurodermatitis, a condition confined to the area at the base of the scalp, characterized by extreme itchiness and common among menopausal and post-menopausal women. Then, there is pityriasis amientacea, a severe form of scaling that usually results in hair loss if left untreated.

Research indicates that dandruff becomes evident when a chemical reaction in the body causes the normal shedding of dead cells to increase, thus making the peeling process, normally imperceptible, much more apparent. Evidence suggests that this chemical change is associated with one or a combination of factors, namely a dietary deficiency, stress, and ill-usage of hair preparations. It goes without saying that dandruff that is obvious is Nature's cry for help!

If a dietary deficiency is likely, eating wholefoods high in vitamins, minerals and trace elements is the best way of correcting it, but it is interesting to note that an undersupply of either the A, B_6 or C vitamins produces various symptoms including common dandruff and seborrhoeaic dermatitis, which is dandruff in a more extreme form.

Dandruff sufferers should begin by following these few dietary rules:

Do
- Eat small quantities of first-class protein-packed foods such as chicken, liver, or another lean meat, fish (white, non-oily kinds), eggs and cottage cheese every day.
- Eat a minimum of one green salad, consisting of pepper, endive, lettuce, watercress, chicory, cabbage, and parsley etc., daily.
- Eat at least two pieces of fruit a day, one of which should be an orange. Choose from apples, grapefruits and pineapples but avoid bananas
- Drink a minimum of six glasses of water daily, beginning with one first thing in the morning
- Take one teaspoonful of brewer's yeast three times a day
- Take 200iu of vitamin E tablets (avoid capsules or wheatgerm oil) daily

Don't
- Eat animal fats (full-fat milk, cheese with a high fat content, butter, cream, ice-cream, pork, bacon, and other fatty meats containing saturated hidden fats), oily fish, or fried, oily or processed foods
- Eat hot-tasting 'spicy' foods
- Eat nuts, avocados and bananas
- Eat salt, sugar, chocolate or pastries

Now that steps have been taken towards improving the diet, try to adopt a positive attitude to stress. Obviously, it is difficult when weighed down by worries, but they are part of life and it is the way we deal with them that ultimately determines the effect, if any, on health (see page 90).

A scalp that has dandruff is sensitive and as such must be treated gently but firmly. Use a gentle shampoo and dilute it before use. Commercial anti-dandruff shampoos in the main are too harsh, but despite warnings about them in *The British Medical Journal* way back in 1956, they continue to be used. Using a dilution of a mild shampoo, apply it in the normal way. Massage gently and rinse until no trace of shampoo remains. Before shampooing, use the Anti-Dandruff Pre-Shampoo Lotion on page 135.

Psoriasis

Psoriasis causes sufferers a great deal of distress because it is not always confined to the scalp. It is difficult to treat, the red patches covered with silver-white scales stubbornly adhering to the scalp and other affected areas. This condition can be hereditary but it is usually stress-related, appearing when resistance is low, and it can also be a reaction to certain foods. There are a number of herbal remedies reputed to cure a variety of skin disorders including psoriasis, but I would urge sufferers to consult their doctor or a trichologist without delay.

DOS AND DON'TS OF WASHING, CONDITIONING AND OTHER HAIR CARE

Do
- Use either a shower or a hand spray attachment to the bath to wash and rinse hair. With bath washing, kneel and bend over the bath to ensure thorough washing and rinsing
- Select a natural shampoo or a vegetable-based one, and dilute it before use
- Pre-rinse hair before applying the shampoo, thus necessitating only the minimum of shampoo
- Pour shampoo (and conditioner too) from the bottle into the palm of the hand, and rub both hands together before working it through the hair. Never apply shampoo or conditioner from the bottle straight on to the hair
- Use only the minimum of shampoo. If hair hasn't been washed for several days, give it a second wash, again using as little shampoo as possible
- Shampoo and rinse with warm, not hot water
- Rinse hair longer than you feel is necessary. When you are certain no traces of shampoo remain, rinse again to be certain
- Use a conditioner every time you wash your hair
- Deep condition once or twice a week if hair is very dry, using the warm oil treatment
- Rinse conditioner out of the hair in the same way as shampoo
- After rinsing out all traces of conditioner, restore the hair's acid mantle by adding one-third of a cup of cider vinegar (for brunettes) or lemon juice for blondes to the final rinse water
- Blot and pat hair dry; don't rub it
- Use a wide-toothed comb with no rough or sharp edges. Avoid metal or other combs with teeth that are sharp
- Remove tangles by combing the hair from the ends upwards while hair is damp
- Brush hair gently but never when wet

- Buy a hair brush made from natural bristle. It's an investment
- Change your style occasionally, or at least part it differently, to give hair a treat
- Always keep hair covered with a scarf in hot or very cold weather, otherwise it may become dry and brittle
- Use the Slant-Board Relaxer every day to promote a good flow of blood to the scalp
- Remember that hair six inches long is about one year old at the ends, and has been subjected to fifty-two shampoos, possibly more, approximately three-hundred and sixty-five brushings and more than two thousand combings, so be kind

Don't
- Allow hair to become dirty before washing it
- Use a shampoo containing sulphur or any anti-dandruff shampoos for dry hair. If hair is dry, include more good quality vegetable oils in the diet. If dandruff is a problem, keep off salt, sugar and oily foods like pork, bacon, nuts, butter, cream, cheese and whole milk
- Use dry shampoos
- Use a shampoo or a massage brush that will snarl and break the hair
- If you have shoulder-length or very long hair, don't pile it on top of your head and rub it as if you are doing the laundry, or it will tangle
- Wait for hair damage before using a conditioner
- Use too much conditioner unless hair tangles easily
- Rub conditioner into the scalp. Conditioner is for the hair
- Leave split ends untreated, or they will get worse
- Use a hair drier too hot, too long, or too often. Far better to let the hair dry naturally
- Use hot curlers, but if you must, wrap tissue on the edge of the hair before rolling
- Brush hair when wet
- Rub, drag, pull or twist hair or it will break
- Wear tight hats or wigs – hair needs to breathe
- Use elastic bands on hair

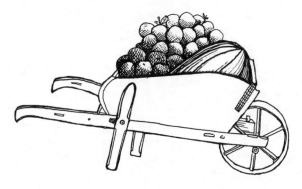

NATURAL HAIR PREPARATIONS

Natural Herbal Shampoo

1lb (450 grams) soft green soap or soft soap BPC
3 pints (1.7 litres) boiling water
4 tablespoons dried rosemary

Pour the boiling water over the rosemary and leave to infuse. Several hours later, strain the herbal liquid into a stainless steel or an aluminium saucepan. Add the soap and bring to the boil over a low heat. Leave the mixture to simmer gently until the soap has dissolved completely. Remove from the heat and when the liquid is cool, pour the clear liquid at the top into a bottle and label. The sediment at the bottom can be thrown away.

Protein-Rich Pre-Shampoo Conditioner

2½ tablespoons dried milk
1 tablespoon wheatgerm oil
1 egg

Whip all the ingredients together until smooth. Apply evenly and gently along the hair. Leave for one hour, preferably longer, before shampooing in the usual way.

An excellent pre-shampoo conditioner for adding lustre and bounce to 'tired' hair.

Pre-Shampoo Conditioner for Dry and Brittle Hair

Castor oil

Pour the oil into a saucepan and heat slowly until nicely warm. Using the finger tips, not the nails, massage the oil gently from the scalp along the hair to the ends. Wrap hair in a nice, warm towel and leave for three hours. Later, gently comb and then wrap the hair in another warm towel, and leave for as long as possible, preferably overnight, before shampooing.

Honeyed Pre-Shampoo Conditioner

4 tablespoons olive oil
2 tablespoons honey

Pour the ingredients into a glass jar with a screw-type lid and shake vigorously until well blended. Leave the mixture to steep for three or four days, giving the jar a good shake whenever you pass. Before shampooing, rub this conditioner liberally into the roots, working along the hair to the ends. Next, comb the hair thoroughly to ensure that the conditioner is evenly distributed. Now, wrap the hair in a large piece of polythene, and leave for one hour, preferably longer. Later shampoo, two light washes being better than one, and rinse thoroughly.

This conditioner is wonderful for revitalizing dull, tired hair and leaves it glossy and manageable.

Anti-Dandruff Pre-Shampoo Lotion

Pour the two liquids into a bottle, shake well and label.

Soak a swab of cotton wool in the solution and dab it on the scalp until the entire area has been treated. Leave for one hour, more if possible, before shampooing the hair in the normal way.

2 fl oz (70ml) Listerine antiseptic
¼ pint (140ml) water (distilled)

Anti-Dandruff Nettle Rub

Pour the boiling water over the nettles, cover, and leave to infuse for three to four hours. Strain, bottle, and label.

This nettle rub can be used as a final rinse after shampooing, or rubbed on to the scalp nightly. This herbal rub helps to combat dandruff, even stubborn cases, when used regularly. A friend of mine who had a bad case of dandruff, having tried what seemed like every anti-dandruff treatment on the market to no avail, asked my advice. I recommended that he use this nettle rub night and morning, which he did, and within a week there were definite signs of improvement. After a couple of months, the dandruff had completely disappeared, leaving his hair shining and healthy. Used regularly, it also helps to promote and strengthen hair growth.

1 handful nettles
2 pints (1.15 litres) boiling water

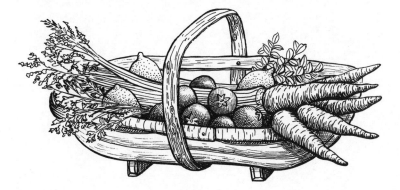

9

Breasts

A BEAUTIFUL BUSTLINE

The breasts are mammary glands cushioned by adipose tissue (fat) and surrounded by fibrous connective tissue. These tissues, along with the genetic 'blueprint' in each of us determine the ultimate size, shape and firmness of the breasts.

Other factors that affect size, though not always for the better, are hormonal changes within the body that result from taking the 'Pill', or undergoing oestrogen treatment for menopausal problems. Consequently, women may experience breast growth which, in some cases, remains, even after discontinuing the treatment.

Drastic weight loss also affects the breasts but not in the way one might expect. Weight loss that occurs suddenly after illness or intensive dieting, particularly if the diet is deficient in vitamin C and other nutrients necessary in the production and maintenance of healthy collagen fibres, can result in sagging breasts that could have been avoided had the weight loss been gradual. A diet high in carbohydrate and low in protein can also have the same effect.

Yet another factor that contributes to sagging breasts is frequent hot baths. To prevent this, always take a warm, not a hot bath and finish off with a cool or cold water splash (see Bathing page 160).

If you want a bust to be proud of, above all watch your posture. Stand sideways in front of a full-length mirror, and check that your back is straight and your shoulders back. You'll find that standing straight lifts your bustline by several inches.

EXERCISES

If your breasts have a tendency to sag, exercise can help considerably. Exercise can't firm the breasts themselves because they have no actual muscles, but it does stimulate the circulation and strengthen the powerful pectoral or chest muscles supporting the breasts which, in turn, tones and lifts sagging breasts.

Swimming, particularly the breast stroke, is an easy and pleasant way of toning and firming up supportive muscles of breasts and upper arms. Here are some other simple exercises to try:

Exercise 1
Kneel on the floor so that your body from your knees upwards is upright. Raise your arms above your head. Press your hands together and gradually increase the pressure and count to five. Now, hold the pressure, count to three and relax. Repeat seven times. This exercise is a great 'up-lifter'.

Exercise 2
Grip your forearms tightly with your hands as if you are about to push up your sleeves. Push towards the elbows without relaxing your grip and relax. Repeat five times. Next, lift the arms to eye level, grip the forearms and push and relax as before. Repeat five times. Finally, lift your arms above your head, and gripping your forearms, push and relax. Repeat five times.

As you feel the muscles tightening, so you can see the breasts lifting. An extremely good exercise for expectant mothers who want to prevent breasts sagging after pregnancy, but you don't need to be pregnant to benefit from this exercise.

Exercise 3
Standing upright, push your arms straight out in front of you with your palms facing the floor. With your arms still outstretched, move them backwards as far as they will go, while pushing out your chest as far as possible without straining. Repeat ten times.

If the exercise is done correctly, you will feel the strong pull of the pectorals with each movement.

Exercise 4
The next two exercises produce faster results when you hold a small weight, such as a book in each hand. I use two jars filled with dry beans, which at 2 lb (1 kg) each is about right. Holding the weights, push your arms straight out in front of you and hold for two seconds. Then, with the arms still outstretched, push them upwards towards the ceiling. Repeat seven times.

This exercise is wonderful for strengthening the pectoral muscles that support the breasts.

Exercise 5
Stand with your feet apart and a weight in each hand. Raise your arms sideways until they are level with your shoulders and begin to make circles in the air. Begin with small ones and gradually let the circles grow larger and larger. Always ensure that the circle drawing of one hand matches the other.

TIPS TO IMPROVE YOUR CLEAVAGE

- Try this tip used by models to give an instant cleavage to plunge-front dresses. Cut several lengths of Sellotape in readiness. Holding the breast in the desired position with one hand, secure the tape to the skin just beneath the breast around the outer curve until it feels adequately supported. Now repeat the process the other side.
    This tip provides the uplift necessary to small bosoms that are not as firm as they once were.
- Emphasize cleavage or create the illusion of one with a subtle application of blusher. Using a tawny shade, brush lightly between breasts until a realistic effect is achieved.
- Highlight an attractive cleavage by applying a blusher sparingly to the curves of the breasts. Select a gold shade with a frosted or a metallic finish.

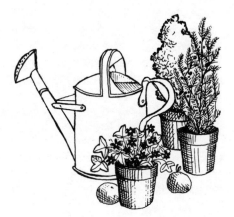

10
Hands and Nails

REVEALING HANDS

Hands are very expressive and reveal a lot about you and your health. A firm handshake is considered a sign of good character, but it also indicates rude health as do warm hands, whereas palms that sweat excessively are associated with anxiety and nervousness. To the trained observer, the way we actually move our hands signals immediate intentions and reveals character far more than the face. We may conceal our emotions behind a mask of indifference, but our hands give us away every time.

To a doctor, nails are a good indicator of a patient's general health. All too often flaking, peeling nails are the result of detergent and other solvent abuse, but a protein or a vitamin A deficiency may be responsible. Most of us suffer from brittle nails at some time or another, but when accompanied by longitudinal ridging they are a typical symptom of anaemia. Other physical conditions – eczema, psoriasis, rheumatism, heart disease, endocrine disturbance and vitamin and mineral deficiencies for example – also produce ridges, furrows and other tell-tale signs that affect the appearance of the nails. Illness, stress, inadequate diet and irresponsible dieting are also associated with poor nail growth. Obviously, an observant fortune teller who knows her job doesn't need the advantage of 'second sight' to tell of a recent illness. She only has to examine her client's nails!

As you can see, hands and nails and their defects reveal a great deal. Yet, despite this fact, hands are still one of the most abused and neglected parts of the body. Often, we fail to realize until it is too late that hands age more rapidly than the face because the skin covering the hands has relatively few oil cells. Consequently, neglected hands are extremely difficult to rejuvenate.

139

A diet recommended for the complexion that is high in brewer's yeast, blackstrap molasses, raw vegetables and fruit, with sufficient quality protein, also helps to keep hands nourished from the inside, but the solution to excessive dryness caused by water, soaps, detergents, household chemicals and extreme temperatures, is in preventive care.

PREVENTIVE CARE

- Always wear gloves, different ones to suit different jobs, for washing-up, housework, gardening, cleaning the car, bathing the dog and other domestic chores
- Cream hands regularly throughout the day and before going to bed
- Treat hands with consideration

There are a variety of hand creams for different jobs. The nourishing creams are greasy and need to be massaged well into the skin. They are efficient and best used at night when a pair of cotton gloves can be worn to ensure maximum absorption. I find that night creams that are too thick or 'tacky' for the face are particularly nourishing to the hands. Barrier creams contain silicone, are water-resistant and provided they are used in accordance with the manufacturer's instructions provide the protection necessary for really rough and dirty jobs. Sunscreens, though not specifically designed for hands, screen hands from the ultra-violet rays that are responsible for cellular damage and unsightly skin blemishes. Finally, there are the fine, non-greasy lotions, such as glycerine and rosewater, simple formulas popular in our grandmothers' day, which should be used lavishly and regularly throughout the day.

Additional preventive care which hands really appreciate:

- Always wear gloves or mittens outside during the cold months, thus preventing poor circulation, chapping and other problems caused by extreme cold
- Wash hands in warm, not hot water; the latter tends to destroy growing cells below the epidermis
- Use as little soap as possible. All soaps, however mild, have a drying effect on the skin
- Always dry hands thoroughly, particularly between the fingers and under rings where skin disease and chapping may occur

NAIL NUTRITION

The nails are composed of keratin, a tough, fibrous protein produced by the cells underneath the cuticle at the base of the nail (the matrix), the exposed part of which is generally referred to as the 'half moon'. Nails grow at the rate of about 1/250 of an inch per day, which is about one-third to one-half as fast as that of the hair.

Generally, growth is quicker in summer than in winter and quickest of all between the ages of eighteen and twenty-eight; nevertheless, these are not the prime factors that ultimately determine growth rate. For strength and flexibility, nails depend on good health and protection from external damage. Growth can actually slow down or stop altogether when the diet is inadequate. Since nails consist mainly of protein, this nutrient along with vitamin A, B complex and other vitamins, minerals and trace elements, particularly, iron, zinc, iodine, sulphur, calcium and potassium, essential to nail development, must be adequate to maintain their health and strength.

Despite claims by cosmetic companies, nail creams and hardeners, in my opinion, are not the solution to brittle nails. The only nail hardeners that really work are the nutrients in the foods we eat. Like most women, I have had difficulties with flaking, brittle nails that bend back leading to painful splitting high up the cuticle. Gelatine was recommended to me in my teens, a popular myth that proclaimed a packet of gelatine a day keeps broken nails at bay. In fact, far from being a protein of high quality, gelatine contains only half the eight amino acids considered essential to human metabolism, and as such, is regarded as a protein of poor quality with few nutritional benefits. Another misconception was that calcium produced strong, healthy nails. I agree that calcium is important and should not be ignored, but nails are composed of protein not calcium and therefore it is protein that is needed to restore nails. I have applied iodine, so-called 'protein creams', hardeners and every conceivable nail treatments dreamed up by the cosmetic companies, and although some helped, none really worked for me.

Where nutrition is concerned, I believe that you are what you eat. In other words, the foods eaten today will make the person of tomorrow. Consequently, I decided that the solution to my nail problems lay in my diet. As you would expect, my daily intake consists of protein of high quality, fresh fruits, plenty of raw vegetables, molasses, wheatgerm and brewer's yeast supplemented with still more vitamins and minerals. My protein intake would put most dieticians to shame, indeed, many would consider it excessive. My liquid intake is also high and consists primarily of milk (skimmed), water, fresh fruit and vegetable juices with the occasional cup of tea or coffee. I considered the possibility of a deficiency but try as I might, I couldn't find one. As time passed and work increased, my nail problems were temporarily forgotten. During a particularly busy period, when I began drinking milk by the glassful, resulting in my milk consumption increasing from one to nearly three pints (1.7 litres) a day, my nails began growing noticeably faster and stronger. As the months passed, and the growth and the condition of the nails improved considerably, I decided that milk and the nutrients it contains were just what my fingernails needed. Knowing the nutritional needs of nails, let us see how milk compares:

A cup of milk (skimmed) contains:

Protein	— 8 grams
Vitamin A	— 500iu
B_1	— 0.09mg
B_2	— 0.4mg
B_3	— 0.21mg
B_6	— 0.102mg
B_{12}	— 0.871mcg
Folic acid	— 12mcg
C	— 2.3mcg
D	— 3.4iu
E	— 0.1mg
Calcium	— 291mg
Iron	— 0.12mg
Phosphorus	— 228mg
Sodium	— 120mg
Potassium	— 370mg
Magnesium	— 33mg

Multiply this by the number of cups consumed daily and its value as a nail food is evident.

I am not asking you to put faith in milk alone, but to increase your intake of eggs, yogurt, cottage cheese and other complete protein foods, which contain all the amino acids, the building blocks for strong, new nail tissue. My finger nails are testimony to the fact that nutritional requirements vary from one individual to the next. Despite my high intake of proteins, it obviously wasn't adequate for all my bodily requirements. Consequently, it is necessary to find the level of protein that is sufficient for you.

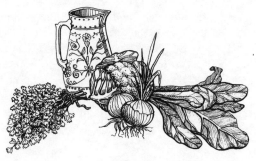

PROBLEMS AND SOLUTIONS

Red, Raw-Looking Hands

For quick relief, mix the juice of an orange with a teaspoonful of honey and apply to the hands.

Rough, Cracked Hands

A combination of drying substances, cold weather and rough jobs are to blame. Rub a wedge of lemon juice over the skin to clean and soften before massaging olive oil well into the hands. Rinse with lukewarm water. Follow with another massage using petroleum jelly. Apply more olive oil and petroleum jelly a few hours later if necessary.

Calluses

Smooth away hard skin with a pumice stone. Rub a slice of lemon over the hands and while still wet, apply handcream lavishly.

Brown Spots on Hands

Check that your diet is balanced and well supplied with B complex, particularly niacin and folic acid. Protect hands from the ultraviolet rays of the sun by applying a high protection sunscreen that is free of bergamot oil.

Blue-Tinged Hands

This is a sign of poor circulation. Keep hands warm by wearing gloves in cold weather. Regular massage will also boost circulation.

Enlarged Veins on the Backs of the Hands

It is the pull of gravity that makes veins fill up with blood and appear so prominent. Lifting hands high in the air makes the veins contract and appear less noticeable.

Stained Fingers and Nails

Bleach away stains by applying freshly squeezed lemon juice on a brush to fingers and nails.

Slow Nail Growth

Exercise your hands and finger-tips to stimulate nail growth. Typing, piano playing, knitting, drumming fingers on a table and massaging the fingers towards the tips encourages circulation to the finger-tips and brings nourishment to the matrix of the nails. Shaking out your hands, and opening and closing quickly outstretched hands also helps stimulate nail growth. Examine your diet to ensure that it is adequately supplied with nail 'foods', particularly protein and vitamin A.

Splitting, Brittle Nails

Such problems are the result of excessive dryness caused by either the over-use of nail polishes, removers, hardeners or soaps or exposure to chlorine, cleaning chemicals or too much sun. Keep nails free of polish, hardeners etc. Correct damage by feeding the matrix with warm oil massages. Check that your diet is adequately supplied with all the nutrients necessary for nail health, particularly protein, vitamin A, B complex and zinc.

White Spots on the Nails

This discolouration can be a sign of illness, stress, a zinc deficiency or the result of injury to the growing nail. Check your diet (see Stress-Reducing Menu on page 92). If a zinc deficiency is suspected, take a zinc supplement (100mg) each day. If it is simply the result of injury, it will grow out in time.

Horizontal Ridges in Nails

This uneven growth is due to either illness or injury to the base of the nail while growing. It will grow out in time. Meanwhile, prevent further re-occurrence by treating cuticles with care.

Blood Spot under a Nail

This damage occurs when a nail becomes jammed in a door or a drawer. Apply cold compresses and keep the hand elevated for a short period.

GUYTON'S PROFESSIONAL MANICURE

This manicure can take you up to one hour to begin with, but as you become more proficient, you will be able to do it in far less time. Try and give yourself this manicure once a week.

1 Dissolve old nail enamel with a wad of cotton wool soaked in an oil-based remover: hold it on the nail for a few seconds and wipe the nail clean in one sweep from the base to the tip

2 Filing is an important part of a manicure. See-saw filing, too low at the corners causes nails to peel and split, whereas good filing helps to prevent it. Nails that are damaged or much too long should be trimmed straight across with nail clippers, not scissors. If nails are brittle, keep them short and don't file the corners too low or it will weaken them further. Using the fine side of an emery board, file from side to centre in one direction. Finish off rough edges by bevelling or stroking the nail gently up and down again with the fine side of the emery board

3 Apply cuticle cream, petroleum jelly or vegetable oil and massage well into the cuticles to stimulate growth

4 Soak nails in warm oil – olive, almond, castor, wheatgerm or ground nut are all very beneficial – for fifteen minutes. Dry hands with a towel

5 Gently coax back cuticles with finger tips. Now, using a cotton bud or an orange stick tipped with a whisp of cotton wool, ease back the cuticles gently using circular movements, but don't poke or jab or it may damage the matrix of the nail and result in ridging

6 Don't trim the cuticles if you can avoid it. It can cause infection and encourage tougher, thicker cuticles

7 Massage oil or cream into the hands using firm movements working upwards from the fingers to the wrists

8 Buffing stimulates circulation and is a wonderful treatment for nails. With nails still oily, take a nail buffer or a piece of chamois leather and buff gently in one direction. Spend about one minute on each nail. I prefer oil to buffing paste because frequent use of the latter can actually weaken the nails and should not be used under nail varnish

9 Try to keep the nails free of nail enamel as much as possible. If it is to be used, apply a little polish remover to cotton wool and sweep it over the nails to remove all traces of oil

10 Paint the nails with white iodine to help harden them

11 Apply a layer of base-coat, free of acetone, to prevent colour pigmentation from discolouring the nails

12 Apply varnish in three straight strokes: one down the middle and one either side.

Never put too much varnish on the brush or it will be uneven and take ages to dry. Always apply a minimum of two coats. Once the final layer is dry, apply a top-coat of clear varnish to give it a high-gloss finish and protect against chipping

13 Remove any trace of varnish on surrounding skin with a cotton bud dipped in varnish remover

Tips
- Avoid dark red and pale creamy shades unless nails are perfectly shaped and hands are fairly youthful-looking
- Pale pinks, corals and clear varnish look best on short nails, stubby fingers and old-looking hands
- Paint the whole nails if they are short or small
- Leave a space either side of the nails when applying varnish to make wide nails and short fingers look slimmer and longer

NATURAL HAND AND NAIL PREPARATIONS

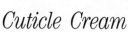

Cuticle Cream

Mix the ingredients together, pot up and label.

4 tablespoons petroleum jelly
1 teaspoon glycerine

Nail Strengthening and Conditioning Oil

Mix the ingredients together, bottle and label. Shake before use. Rub this oil well into the nails before going to bed.

2 tablespoons castor oil
1 tablespoon olive oil

Rosewater Hand Gel

7 tablespoons
rosewater
2 tablespoons
glycerine
2 tablespoons
arrowroot
(powdered)

Pour the rosewater into an enamel bowl and place it in a saucepan of hot water to warm the rosewater ready for use later. Place the glycerine in a separate enamel container and slowly warm over a low heat. Add the arrowroot, a little at a time, stirring the mixture constantly. Finally, add the warm rosewater, remove from the heat and continue to stir until the mixture clears. Pot up, label and refrigerate.

Sunflower Hand Cleanser

1 tablespoon
sunflower oil
1 tablespoon caster
sugar

Mix the ingredients together, pot up and label. Work the cleanser well into the skin and around and under the nails. Rinse off with warm water and pat dry.

I make up a large quantity and keep it in the kitchen so that it is available immediately it is required.

Kaolin Barrier Cream

1 dessertspoon
sunflower oil
1 egg yolk
kaolin powder

Whisk the oil and egg yolk together and add just sufficient powder to transform the yellow liquid into a spreadable paste. This barrier cream should be rubbed on the hands before tackling any dirty jobs.

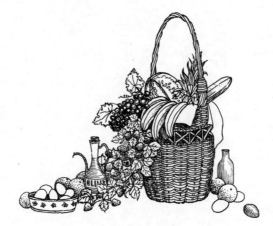

11
Legs

The basic function of human legs throughout Man's evolution was one of mobility and 'flight', and muscles, bones and tendons have all evolved for strength, power, and agility in order to survive. Nowadays, women's legs are admired for their shapeliness, not their muscle-power, and as fashion exposes more of the female leg and ankles, calves, knees and thighs are highlighted, so the imperfections become increasingly apparent.

Genetic factors determine the length and the basic shape of the legs and the thickness of the ankles etc., and no amount of dieting, exercise and massage will change that. Although you can't choose your leg type, you can improve their overall shape and general appearance by diet, exercise, massage and camouflage, but let us begin by considering the problems that mar leg loveliness.

PROBLEMS AND SOLUTIONS

Varicose Veins

Varicose veins are unsightly, unpleasant and potentially dangerous. Occasionally, they are hereditary, like the colour of the hair, and can only be treated surgically, but such cases are rare. Generally, they are caused by an overloading of the veins, due to a weakness in the vein walls, or a malfunction of the blood vessels in the legs.

This condition is common among Western people whose diet is high in refined foods, but relatively unknown among people in less developed societies who live on unrefined foods consisting of wholegrains, raw vegetables, and other foods high in fibre and vitamins C and E. Once you have varicose veins it is difficult to get rid of them except by surgery or injection, and daily rest is an essential part of the treatment.

Obviously prevention is far easier than treatment and so to ensure that you don't get varicose veins, a) follow a high-fibre, low-carbohydrate diet, b) increase your intake of vitamins C and E, the former helping to keep veins strong and healthy and the latter for dilating arteries and increasing circulation, c) don't let yourself become overweight, d) take plenty of exercise (swimming, walking and dancing are particularly good because they strengthen muscles and improve circulation to the lower limbs), and e) don't stand about for long periods, but if it can't be avoided, try to put your feet up regularly every hour or whenever you can.

Studies have shown that nutritional supplements, using vitamin C with its anti-inflammatory quality and its ability to keep veins healthy, and vitamin E that dissolves clots and boosts circulation, are helpful not only in preventing but in treating varicosity.

Adelle Davis in her book *Let's Eat Right to Keep Fit*, recalls the case of a young woman and keen tennis player who developed huge, unsightly varicose veins in pregnancy and whose doctor told her that she could never play tennis again. Miss Davis goes on to say:

'At the seventh month a marble-sized purple clot appeared near the skin, causing her entire leg to become inflamed and continuously painful. Her doctor kept her in bed, urged her to allow labour to be induced, and told her that surgery would be necessary. At this point she started taking 300 units of vitamin E after each meal; and because of the inflammation, she also took 1000 milligrams of vitamin C six times daily. This girl and her mother both declared that not only the clot but also the varicose veins disappeared before their eyes. A week after her delivery, she was again playing tennis, her legs having become completely normal.'

Thread (Spider) Veins

Broken, surface capillaries that appear as spidery, purplish veins on thighs, behind knees and around ankles are unattractive but not dangerous, and as such, are a cosmetic rather than a health problem. In serious cases where they are obvious and cause embarrassment, they can be treated by schlerotherapy, which involves injecting a chemical into the tiny veins that dries up the blood and makes them disappear. Mild cases can be camouflaged with make-up and dark-toned stockings. Increased intakes of vitamin C help strengthen the capillary walls and thus minimize further rupturing.

Swollen Legs and Ankles

Temporary swelling of the legs and/or the ankles, characterized by a swollen area that when pressed leaves a small depression that slowly disappears, is caused by standing too long. As a result, body fluids in the blood leach out of the veins and arteries into the surrounding tissues and make the area swell. If this occurs and you happen to be overweight or pregnant, rest your legs by putting them up, or better still, raising them above your head, and here the Slant-Board Relaxer is extremely beneficial.

Many women in their late thirties and early forties complain of swollen legs, particularly around the ankles, prior to menstruation. To control this, one must minimize fluid retention by a) reducing salt intake, which causes water retention and b) eating more foods that have diuretic properties – cucumber and celery are two of the best natural diuretics known – and drinking a combination of cucumber, cabbage and grapefruit juice, by blending together all the ingredients with water in a liquidizer.

Finally, bathing the ankles and legs in warm, not hot water containing epsom salts and massaging the legs from the feet upwards towards the thighs, using smooth strokes, also brings relief.

Scorch Marks

Scorch marks, caused by sitting too near a fire, are not as common as they once were. The damage occurs usually below the horny layer of dead cells at the epidermis, and time is needed for the top layer of skin to peel off before exposing the damaged cells below, which, in turn, have to flake off before new, unscarred skin is visible. The natural flaking process can be speeded up by exfoliation, which involves rubbing a handful of dry salt or moistening oatmeal (fine) over wet legs. Meanwhile, the discolouration can be lightened slightly by applying a dilution of lemon juice and water, but several applications are necessary.

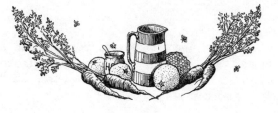

EXERCISE

Legs need exercise and plenty of it daily to keep them in shape, tone and good condition. Here are some exercises designed specifically to trim and firm, improve overall shape and keep circulation at a high level.

Exercise 1 (for the whole leg)
Standing with your feet parallel and your arms in front, bend the knees, keeping the heels on the floor. On the third bend, raise your heels and bend right down to a crouching position. Now rise slowly counting to five. Repeat five times.

Exercise 2 (for inner thighs)
Sit on the floor on your side so that your elbows are supporting your weight. Keeping your legs straight with one resting on top of the lower one, slowly raise and lower your legs. Repeat ten times. Now repeat the exercise on the other side.

Exercise 3 (for thighs and hips)
Lie back on the floor with your arms outstretched and one knee bent. Lift the other leg and with the knee straight, make large, sweeping circles in the air. The wider the circles, the better the exercise. Do ten circles with one leg in a clockwise direction and another ten in an anti-clockwise direction. Repeat with the other leg.

Exercise 4
Kneel on the floor with your back straight and your arms outstretched in front of you at shoulder level. Keeping your body in a straight line, slowly lean backwards as far as possible without straining or falling. Now slowly return to your original, vertical position. As thighs become stronger, so you will be able to stretch further with relative ease. Repeat eight times.

Exercise 5 (knees)
Kneel with your legs flat on the floor. Now take a deep breath and arch your body backwards and grip your ankles with your hands. Hold to a count of four and return to your original position. Repeat six times.

Exercise 6 (for knees and calves)
Sit on the floor with your legs outstretched in a wide V. Now, bending your knees slightly, draw your heels in towards you. Next, stretch your legs and knock the backs of your knees against the floor twice. Finally, bring your legs together straight in front of you and knock the backs of the knees against the floor twice. Repeat eight times.

Exercise 7 (for calves and ankles)
Stand with your heels on the floor and your toes resting on an ordinary telephone directory (not Yellow Pages which is far too thick). Lift yourself on to your toes, hold to a count of ten and return to your original position. Repeat five times.

Exercise 8 (for calves and ankles)
Standing upright, walk across the room on tip-toe. Now, still on your toes, walk backwards into the room.

Exercise 9 (for calves and ankles)
Standing upright, stand on tip-toe as high as you can. Hold to a count of six and relax. Repeat ten times.

Exercise 10 (for ankles)
Sit on a chair and cross your legs. With the toes of the top foot pointing upright in the air, slowly rotate the ankle, twelve times in a clockwise direction and twelve times in an anti-clockwise direction. Repeat with the other ankle.

TIPS FOR SMOOTH, LOVELY LEGS

- Keep legs hair-free by regularly shaving or using depilatory creams, waxes or abrasive gloves
- Use a loofah or friction mitt in circular movements on rough 'chicken' skin. On stubborn patches where nothing seems to help, soak in an oil bath for twenty minutes (see Bathing, page 160). Afterwards, pat dry, and massage the problem area with petroleum jelly, removing any excess with tissues
- Tone, stimulate and exfoliate the skin regularly in the bath, by taking a handful of fine seasalt and gently rubbing it all over the legs using circular movements
- Apply a moisturizer to the legs daily, preferably after a bath while the skin is still damp. Massage body lotion or hand cream in smooth, upward strokes from ankle to knee and from knee to thigh
- If the legs are on the 'chunky' side, wear dark brown or grey tone stockings with dark shoes and a skirt or a dress to match that comes below the knees, so that you create the illusion of a long, slim line from waist to toe
- If you have well-developed calf muscles, avoid certain sports, particularly bicycling which is a real calf-developer!
- Unless you have plump legs or wish to camouflage marks on them, wear sheer ten or fifteen denier tights or stockings

- Don't cross your legs high up so that one thigh is resting on the other, for by doing so, you are impeding the blood flow, which could lead to thick thighs and circulatory problems
- Walk tall and straight. Whatever their shape, legs look best when you walk straight with your feet parallel and toes pointing forward
- Stimulate leg muscles by varying the height of your heel throughout the day, by keeping two extra pairs of shoes at the office of different heel heights from each other and from the pair you wear to work

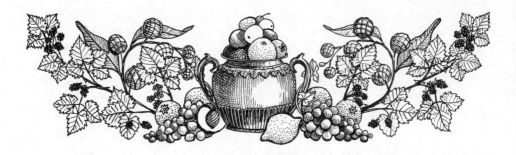

12
Feet

The human foot is the most remarkable example of anatomical engineering. Each consists of twenty-six small, delicate bones, the highest concentration of bone in the body, with over two hundred ligaments and twenty muscles that contain, support and cushion the bones and joints and lend flexibility to the foot. Together, they bear and balance our entire body weight in every step we take and for a town dweller, who walks perhaps an average seven to ten miles a day, that is an awful lot of steps.

Yet, this perfect structure, designed to enable us to walk, run, grip and balance freely is encased in socks, tights or stockings made of man-made fibres, pushed into restrictive footwear that is shaped to accommodate fashion rather than feet, and forced to pound hard floors and pavements. Despite the fact that we will probably walk a minimum of 100,000 miles in our lifetime, feet are given little more than the most cursory attention until they begin to hurt. Then, the pain registers in our face and posture. But we don't need to see our pained reflection to know the effect the shoes are having on our feet. The corns, blisters and calluses speak for themselves. Heels that are too high throw the balance of the body out of alignment resulting in pain, backache, leg problems and fatigue. We are all painfully familiar with ill-fitting shoes and the damage they cause, so don't buy a pair, however attractive they are, unless they feel just right in every way. Remember, shoes that don't fit properly will always be uncomfortable.

My own remedy for painful feet is water and walking on tip-toe. It sounds a strange combination but there is nothing quite like it to strengthen tired feet. Try it in your home or in the garden on a nice, springy lawn. Remove shoes and stockings and walk bare-foot on your toes, as if you are dancing, for five minutes. Then, place a chair near the bath and sit on it with your legs dangling into the bath. Let warm water from the mixer-tap or shower flow over your feet for two minutes, followed by cold water for one minute.

155

This therapeutic treatment takes only eight minutes in total to completely strengthen and revitalize tired and painful feet.

FOOT REVIVERS

- Rub an ice cube over hot, swollen feet to soothe and refresh them
- Relax tired feet by using the Slant-Board Relaxer (see page 91)
- If your feet are really 'killing you', soak them in a bowl of warm water containing a handful of either sea salt or baking soda, or a mixture consisting of one tablespoonful each of borax and epsom salts
- Rev-up sore, aching feet with a friction rub. Apply surgical spirit or cider vinegar to a piece of coarse linen and rub it all over the feet
- Sprinkle alum powder on the feet when they feel sore and tired. It will soothe and harden them up extremely well
- Slough off old skin once a week by rubbing a handful of coarse salt on to the feet, concentrating particularly on the soles and backs of the feet

PROBLEMS AND SOLUTIONS

Corns

Corns are the foot's way of protecting itself from friction and pressure that result from poorly fitting shoes. Soak feet in warm salty water for fifteen minutes and then use a pumice stone to rub away small, soft corns. Large corns should be removed professionally by a qualified chiropodist. Meanwhile, a padded ring designed for the purpose can be worn over the corn to relieve pressure. Don't attempt to remove it yourself with a knife or razor blade or you will risk injury or infection.

Calluses

A callus is an area of hard skin caused by ill-fitting shoes. Although less painful than a corn, it can produce a tender, burning sensation that makes walking difficult. Soak your feet in warm water and then smooth the hard tissue with a pumice stone or foot scraper before massaging lanolin, castor oil or petroleum jelly into the feet. An area that is thickly callused will require several treatments.

Bunions

A bunion is a thickening of the skin at the head of the metatarsal bone that manifests itself as a hard, unsightly and sometimes painful swelling over the joint at the base of the big toe. It may be the result of tight stockings, or small or narrow shoes, but in many cases it is a hereditary weakness in the foot construction that puts the foot out of alignment. If professional help is sought in the early stages, it may be possible to treat it with corrective exercises, but when fully developed, surgery may be the only answer. Women who have undergone this operation admit that it is a painful experience, particularly when attempting to walk again.

Verrucas

These are viral infections that appear as inward-growing warts which are painful when pressure is applied. They can appear singly or in clusters. If they are covered with a ring of felt to relieve the pressure, they can clear-up by themselves. Failing this, they must be removed by a chiropodist.

Athlete's Foot

This fungal disease, so called because athletes run the risk of contracting it by going barefoot in gyms, public showers and swimming pools, thrives on warm, damp skin, and is highly contagious. It usually appears between the toes as scaly flakiness and spreads quickly to the soles and other parts of the feet, resulting in itchy skin that cracks and is extremely painful. Always wash feet after going barefoot in any public place and dry them thoroughly. Keep feet as dry, clean and fresh as possible and change tights and socks daily. There are a variety of preparations in both liquid and powder form to treat this infection, but if it persists, consult a doctor or a chiropodist.

Ingrowing Toenails

The problem of the sides of the toenails growing into the skin is caused by cutting the nails down at the sides instead of straight across. It must be treated professionally, as early as possible, as it can be difficult to remedy if left. Some ingrowing toenails remain painful for life simply because they were not treated by a chiropodist at the onset. Don't try to cut the nail free or you risk inflammation and might make it even more difficult to treat.

Chilblains

Poor circulation is to blame for the inflamed and painful condition known as chilblains. The nutritional approach is to increase the intake of vitamins that boost circulation, such as niacin in a B complex formula and vitamin E. Improving the circulation further by a) exercising, b) massaging and c) plunging the feet in cold water for thirty seconds and wearing a pair of woollen socks afterwards is also very beneficial. Wear socks, clothing, shoes and boots made of natural fibres that are neither too tight nor too small and don't restrict circulation.

PEDICURE

1 Remove nail enamel by pressing cotton wool soaked in oily remover on the nail for a second or two and wipe off
2 Soak feet in warm water in which is dissolved sea salt or any other foot reviver, for

ten minutes. Use a bristle brush to scrub the toes, heels and soles of the feet

3   After soaking, plunge the feet into cold water for thirty seconds to boost circulation

4   Use a pumice stone to remove calluses and rough, dry skin

5   Dry feet thoroughly, particular attention being paid between the toes

6   Use a nail clipper to cut the nails in a straight line from corner to corner. Never allow the nails to extend beyond the tip of the toes. Smooth rough edges with an emery board but don't shape the nails

7   Apply oil or cuticle cream to the cuticles and work in. Gently ease back the cuticles and clean the nails and sides with the tip of an orange stick wrapped in cotton wool

8   Check that you haven't missed any hard or 'horny' areas before massaging either foot oil (see below) or hand cream into the feet

9   Buff nails to stimulate circulation. Work in one direction, not back and forth, which overheats the nails

10 If nails are to be varnished, weave a strip of tissue between the toes to prevent the enamel from smudging. Apply base-coat to protect the nails and leave it to dry hard. Apply two coats of nail enamel, allowing each one to dry completely between applications. Avoid bright oranges and reds, particularly purple-reds, and very pale metallic shades. Soft pinks, corals and clear varnishes are far more flattering. Finish off with a clear, protective top-coat

Luxury Foot Oil

Mix the ingredients together, bottle and label. Massage the oil evenly around the toes, soles, heels and ankles and any excess oil can be massaged into the legs to smooth and beautify them. This lovely, musky-smelling oil helps relieve tired and strained feet and keeps them soft and smooth.

10 tablespoons almond oil
12 drops clove oil

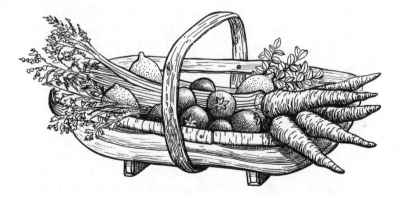

13
Bathing

The weekly bath is a thing of the past. Education and improved bathing facilities have resulted in increased personal hygiene, but bathing is no longer merely a matter of cleansing. Nowadays, with the emphasis on natural ingredients, bathing is also appreciated for its cosmetic and therapeutic value.

Throughout history, many famous beauties have used natural ingredients in the bath to soften and nourish, tone and moisturize the skin, from the legendary Cleopatra who luxuriated in asses' milk to Madame de Pompadour, the beautiful mistress of Louis XV of France who soaked in baths of herbs for long periods every day. Even as early as AD 212, Romans congregated en masse in the elegant and most beautiful of all bath houses, the Caracalla, where they had at least twenty-five different baths from which to choose, the oil bath being a particular favourite among the ladies.

Each time you step into the bath you are joining the esprit de corps of the renowned beauties of the world, from Cleopatra, Madame de Pompadour and Nefertiti, the lovely wife of an Egyptian Pharaoh, to Mumtaz Mahal, whose husband Shah Jehan so adored her that he built the most beautiful of white, marbled mausoleums, the Taj Mahal, in memory of her.

LUXURIOUS BATHS

Oil Bath

Soap is an excellent solvent, but even fairly fatty soaps tend to neutralize the natural oils in the body, which results in dry skin. After a long day when you need to soak and unwind in a warm bath, but have neither the energy nor the inclination to apply a body oil afterwards to counteract the drying effect, take an oil bath.

Whisk the ingredients together, bottle and label. Shake vigorously before use. Add two or three tablespoonfuls to the running water.

This delightful oil treatment coats the body in a fine film, thus helping to retain sebum while moisturizing at the same time. Step out of the bath and massage the oil with a coarse bath towel. The gentle friction will stimulate the circulation, leaving the body toned and feeling soft and silky.

Note: Oil is inclined to make the bath slippery so be careful when stepping in and out.

1 pint (570ml) corn, olive, sesame or sunflower oil
2 tablespoons hair shampoo (ordinary and inexpensive)
1 teaspoon toilet water or eau de cologne

Milk Bath

Of all bathing treatments, the milk bath is the essence of luxury. Unlike Cleopatra, you may not have a herd of asses to supply gallons of fresh milk each day, but fresh and dried cow's milk will do just as well.

Pour the fresh and powdered milk into the bath and swirl the water around until the powder has completely dissolved. Add a few drops of toilet water if desired.

Step into the bath and gently loofah your body using lots of water but no soap. Soak for fifteen minutes.

The milk nourishes and softens rough skin, imparting a glowing, satiny texture to the entire body. Don't soap yourself or the milk and its therapeutic effects will be lost.

1 pint (570ml) fresh milk
8 oz (225 grams) powdered milk
A few drops toilet water (optional)

Seaweed Bath

I always try to gather supplies of fresh seaweed whenever I am by the sea for use in the bath. Rich in iodine, and an excellent source of iron, calcium, sodium, potassium and phosphorus, seaweed baths tone the skin, relax muscles that are tired and tense, and so it is believed, are helpful to slimmers who are fighting the 'flab'. Obviously, it is more convenient to use powdered kelp from a health food shop, but there is nothing like seaweed fresh from the sea.

A few strands fresh or dried seaweed (rinsed and chopped) or 1 tablespoonful powdered kelp

Place the seaweed or the powdered kelp into the foot of an old, clean stocking, cut off at the ankle, and hang it just below the running hot water tap, so that the water is flowing through the 'bag'. When the bath is half to three-quarters filled with hot water, leave the bag to soak for fifteen minutes, by which time the bath water should be comfortably warm.

Step in the bath and loofah your body before soaking in the water for fifteen minutes.

Sea Salt Bath

The finest sea salt bath known to man is the sea itself, so always go for a 'dip' whenever you visit the coast. Sea salt eases muscular strain, and adding it to the bath is a superb way to tone, firm and tighten loose and flabby skin. It also has the advantage of drawing out the toxins from the pores, thus easing and relaxing taut muscles. Salt has a healing yet slightly drying effect so if you have very dry skin, add a little vegetable oil to the salty water.

8 oz (225 grams) sea salt (fine) 2 tablespoonfuls vegetable oil (optional)

Dissolve the salt in the water and add the oil, if necessary. The water should never be hot because of its loosening effect on the skin and muscles and its general drying effect.

Soak in the salty water for up to twenty minutes, depending on your skin type.

Emollient Bath

My maternal grandmother had a smooth, silky, and flawless complexion to the day she died. One of her treatments for maintaining her beautiful skin was the emollient bath which she took twice a week. It is wonderfully relaxing and as its name implies, is a superb skin softener.

½ lb (225 grams) barley meal 1 lb (450 grams) bran ½ oz (12 gram) borax

Put all the ingredients in a saucepan containing four pints of water, cover, bring to the boil, and leave to simmer over a low heat for fifteen minutes. Remove from the heat and let it steep for one hour. Finally, strain the liquid into the bath, half-filled with warm water.

My grandmother always soaked in it for about twenty minutes but by all means luxuriate in it for as long as you wish.

Note: The strained mixture, topped up each time with a small quantity of fresh ingredients, can be re-used several times.

Cider Vinegar Bath

Bathing is a great ally to beauty, but in dissolving dirt, it inadvertently also removes the acid mantle which cloaks and protects the skin. As a result, complexions often feel taut and mask-like after washing. One way to restore the acid balance is to take a cider vinegar bath. It alleviates dryness and itchiness, and soothes, tones and softens the skin at the same time. This beauty bath is also excellent for relieving tired and aching muscles.

Add the vinegar to the bath water, lie back and relax for twenty minutes at least, longer if you wish, at the end of which the tiredness will have disappeared and you will be feeling completely rejuvenated.

½ pint (285ml)
cider vinegar

Herbal Bath

Legend has it that the renowned French beauty, Ninon de Lenclos retained a youthful complexion throughout her long life, and her seemingly ageless beauty was attributed to the herbal mixture added to her bath water. This recipe is almost as famous as the celebrated lady herself.

Place all the ingredients in either a muslin or a cheesecloth bag or the foot of an old stocking. Pour boiling water over the closed bag and let it steep for twenty minutes. Then, add both the infusion and the bag to the bath water.

1 tablespoon mint
1 tablespoon thyme
1 tablespoon rosemary
1 tablespoon lavender
1 tablespoon comfrey root (powdered)

Here are some other herbal bath combinations:
- Chamomile flowers, elderflowers, comfrey and linden blossoms (cleanses and softens)
- Sage, thyme, lavender, marjoram and comfrey leaves (relaxes)
- Mint, basil and rosemary (calms)
- Elderflowers, blackberry leaves and geranium leaves (warms)
- Bay leaves (relieves strained muscles)
- Mint and pine needles (refreshes)
- Eucalyptus and pine needles (relaxes)
- Chamomile, rosemary, horsetail and pine needles (cleanses and stimulates)
- Marigold leaves (heals and soothes)

BODY LOTIONS

Rosewater and Lime Body Lotion

6 tablespoons
rosewater
2 tablespoons lime
juice (fresh)
1 tablespoon
glycerine

Mix the ingredients together, bottle, label and refrigerate.

Unlike body oils, this light and refreshing body lotion is absorbed quickly into the skin. After bathing, massage it into your arms, legs and body.

Strawberry Astringent Body Lotion

½ lb (225 grams)
strawberries
(over-ripe)
½ pint (285ml)
vodka or
industrial alcohol

Place the strawberries in a large jar with a screw-type lid, add the alcohol and seal. Shake the contents several times a day for three days. On the fourth day, strain the liquid into a bottle with a screw-type lid, label and refrigerate.

This delightful astringent, which is the essence in luxury, helps remove discolourations of the skin.

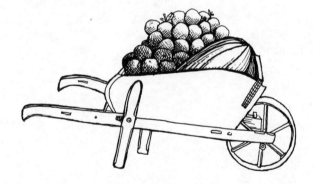

14

Hydrotherapy (Water Treatment)

One of the most potent agents that possesses therapeutic properties capable of age retardation is water.

In Britain and the USA, water is still used primarily for its cleansing qualities and for relaxing tense muscles, but in the health spas and clinics of the world dedicated to rejuvenation and age retardation, men and women wade knee-deep in cool streams and troughs of running water to improve circulation to feet, legs and abdominal muscles and enhance vitality and immunity to disease. Jets of cold water directed on to specific parts of the body are used to treat conditions from arthritis and eczema to diabetes and heart disease. The water cure in all its many forms also reduces the effects of stress, cures insomnia, revitalizes the body and retards premature ageing.

Water therapy began in Bavaria in the 1840s when Sebastian Kneipp, the son of a poor weaver, who was studying for the priesthood, contracted tuberculosis, an incurable disease in those days. Unwilling to accept the prognosis of doctors, which was virtually a death sentence, Kneipp began reading about the curative powers of water and experimenting on himself which, combined with his increasing awareness of the body's own powers of healing and regeneration, resulted in a complete cure. Now utterly convinced that 'water contains great healing powers', Father Kneipp developed a therapeutic and preventive system, which he used to treat increasing numbers of ailing people who were either too poor or too ill for ordinary medical treatment. His unconventional methods and his reputation grew and the tiny village of Worishofen, where he finally settled and practised, mushroomed to become Bad Worishofen, the largest spa in Europe and one devoted entirely to his treatments, to which thousands of people continue to flock annually from all over the world to take a 'Kneippkur'. Kneipp's methods, which have been researched, improved and updated, are practised today in hospitals all over the world to overcome the effects of injury and disease.

BASIC RULES

Hydrotherapy can be enjoyed at home, but to gain the full benefits, one must follow a few basic rules, which are as follows:
- Wait for at least one, preferably two hours after a meal before taking a bath or applying any water treatment to the body
- Avoid cold baths or any water treatments during menstruation that involve the lower part of the body. Treatments must be confined to the upper part of the body
- Never take a cold bath when the body is cold
- Always make sure before taking a bath that the bathroom is nicely warm
- Avoid hot baths of 95°F (35°C) and over; the loosening effect on muscles is contrary to the firming effect required
- Begin by adding cold water to a warm bath until it is cool, thus avoiding an instant low temperature until the system has become acclimatized to cold water treatments
- Always lie down and rest for a minimum of thirty minutes after a warm bath to obtain the full benefits of the treatment
- After a cool bath, warm up quickly by either exercising or resting in a warm bed

SPECIAL TREATMENTS

The Sitz or 'Youth' Bath

The sitz bath is used to relieve stress, piles, constipation and diarrhoea, the uterine diseases peculiar to women and the genital and urinary diseases common to men, but I like it because it boosts immunity, counteracts fatigue and 'peps' you up.

Half-fill the bath with cool (not cold) water and sit in it sideways with your legs dangling over the side, so that the abdomen and lower part of the body are covered. Remain there for between three and five minutes, no longer. Step out and dry yourself before climbing into a warm bed. Once you have taken several cool sitz baths and are used to them, lower the temperature of the water a little each time until you can take a cold one comfortably.

The Barefoot Treatment

Another Kneipp treatment using cold water to produce vital heat to stimulate the circulation and strengthen the immune system.

There are lovely places to walk in Bavaria, but this treatment can be carried out effectively and just as easily in the privacy of your own garden. It involves walking barefoot on grass that is wet from either dew, rain or watering, for between fifteen and forty-five minutes each day. Immediately afterwards, with your feet still wet, put on a pair of dry socks and shoes and go for a ten-minute walk, starting at a brisk pace and gradually slowing down to a more comfortable speed.

Treading Water

Yet another of Kneipp's cures where patients walk barefoot in pools and running streams every day of the year. Those fortunate enough to live by the sea can take a daily 'paddle', but similar results can be achieved by treading a bath of cold water.

Treading water protects against infection and age degeneration, reduces stress and by so doing eases stress-related disorders like headaches and migraines, and practised before going to bed helps those who have difficulty sleeping.

Dressed with only the feet and legs bare from the knee downwards, step into a bath of cold water and walk on the spot, lifting one foot out of the water before putting the other foot forward, as if you are exercising in an exaggerated way on a walking machine. The initial reaction varies from a lovely warm sensation to a cold ache that is followed by warmth. Begin by treading water for about twenty seconds and gradually increase the time to a couple of minutes, as your system becomes acclimatized. Step out and without drying pull on a pair of dry, warm socks and shoes and keep warm by exercising or moving about.

The Blitzguss

A proper Blitzguss is carried out by a professional therapist using a powerful jet of water, but a similar effect can be achieved with a hand-held shower or a shower attachment to the bath. This treatment taken daily increases one's immunity to infection, enhances vitality, and helps to slow down the ageing process, but it should only be taken after the system has been strengthened by other treatments mentioned here.

Begin by taking a warm shower in the normal way and when your skin is pink and warm, turn off the hot-water tap and direct the cold water over your face and down your arms, legs, upper and lower trunk and back. The whole operation should take no longer than thirty seconds. Step out of the bath or shower, pat-off the excess moisture, wrap in a bath robe and keep warm.

The Wechselbad or Alternating Bath

A good way of increasing resistance to infection by stimulating the circulation and a favourite with Gayelord Hauser, a nutritionist who became something of a legend in his lifetime.

Step into a bath of warm water, and after washing, lie back and relax. When you feel calm and refreshed, drain away half of the water before turning on the cold water tap. Mix the cold and warm water together and as the water gets progressively cooler, your body will begin to tingle. After three minutes stand up, towel yourself dry and climb into a warm bed and relax for about half-an-hour.

The Cold 'Blitzguss' Facial

This facial, which consists of a jet of running water directed on to the face, stimulates the blood supply to the skin, thus nourishing, toning and firming loose, sagging skin. A popular and effective treatment for those who wish to prevent facial ageing and so retain a youthful complexion.

An ordinary handshower or cold-water tap must be adapted to produce a jet of fine water, by simply unscrewing the shower nozzle or attaching a length of plastic piping with an aperture of half an inch to the cold tap.

Bending over the bath and holding the hose or hand piece between two and three inches from your face, turn on the cold water so that it flows off the face smoothly without splashing. Begin by directing the water around your face several times. Now direct the jet up and down from one side of your face to the other and back again. Next, move across the face, beginning at the temple and ending across the jawline. Finally, end as you started by circling the face several times. Pat excess moisture with a towel and allow the skin to dry naturally. The whole treatment should only take about a couple of minutes.

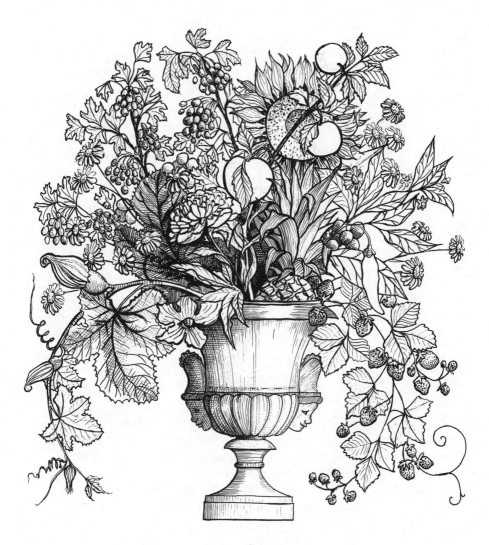

169

Progress Chart

	Day 1	Day 2	Day 3	Day 4	Day 5	Day 6	Day 7	Weekly Total	Weekly Goal
DIET									
Protein:									
Liver, Fish, Chicken, Meat (lean), eggs (per portion)	—	—	—	—	—	—	—	—	7 portions
Vitamins									
A (iu)	—	—	—	—	—	—	—	—	35–70,000iu
B (complex) per tablet	—	—	—	—	—	—	—	—	7–14 tablets
C (mg)	—	—	—	—	—	—	—	—	700–20,000mg
D (iu)	—	—	—	—	—	—	—	—	2,800–4,200iu
E (iu)	—	—	—	—	—	—	—	—	980–2,800iu
Multi-mineral & trace element (tablet)	—	—	—	—	—	—	—	—	7–14 tablets
Supplementary foods per teaspoon:									
Blackstrap molasses	—	—	—	—	—	—	—	—	14 teaspoons
Brewer's yeast	—	—	—	—	—	—	—	—	14–21 teaspoons
Wheatgerm	—	—	—	—	—	—	—	—	21–35 teaspoons
Others:	—	—	—	—	—	—	—	—	—
Liquids (per glass):									
Vegetable juices	—	—	—	—	—	—	—	—	14 glasses
Fruit juices	—	—	—	—	—	—	—	—	14 glasses
Water	—	—	—	—	—	—	—	—	28 glasses
Raw food:									
Salads (per portion)	—	—	—	—	—	—	—	—	7–14 portions
Fruit (each)	—	—	—	—	—	—	—	—	14 pieces (min)
Weight	—	—	—	—	—	—	—	—	see weight chart

	Day 1	Day 2	Day 3	Day 4	Day 5	Day 6	Day 7	Weekly Total	Weekly Goal
EXERCISE (minutes)									
(fast enough to increase heart activity and induce sweating)									
Walking									
or Swimming	—	—	—	—	—	—	—	——	60–210 mins
or Dancing									
or Others									
TREATMENTS (number)									
Skin and Neck (excluding basic cleansing, washing and moisturising)	—	—	—	—	—	—	—	——	7–14 treatments
Hair (excluding shampooing, conditioning (hot oil treatments), setting, drying & colouring)	—	—	—	—	—	—	—	——	2–7 treatments
Hands & Nails (excluding varnishing)	—	—	—	—	—	—	—	——	2–7 treatments
Legs & feet	—	—	—	—	—	—	—	——	2–7 treatments
Bath treatments	—	—	—	—	—	—	—	——	2–7 treatments
Hydrotherapy treatments	—	—	—	—	—	—	—	——	3–7 treatments
SLEEP	—	—	—	—	—	—	—	——	49–56 hours

Index

172

173